KIDNEY STONE DIET COOKBOOK FOR BEGINNERS

Comprehensive Guide to Preventing and Managing Kidney Stones with Easy-to-Follow Recipes, Detailed Nutritional Information, and Lifestyle Tips

Kingsley Klopp

To show our appreciation for your purchase, we're delighted to offer you these special bonuses as a heartfelt thank you.

1. **A Food Tracker Journal**
2. **Downloadable E-BOOK featuring full-color images of finished recipes**

Copyright © 2024 All rights reserved.

No part of this book may be reproduced or transmitted in any form or by any means, electronic or mechanical, including photocopying, recording, or by any information storage and retrieval system, without written permission from the author. The scanning, uploading, and distribution of this book via the internet or via any other means without the permission of the author is illegal and punishable by law. The author has made every effort to ensure the accuracy of the information contained in this book. However, the author cannot be held responsible for any errors or omissions.

Table of Contents

Introduction..7

Chapter 1: Understanding Kidney Stones
- What are Kidney Stones?..9
- Types of Kidney Stones...10
- Causes and Risk Factors...12

Chapter 2: Basics of the Kidney Stone Diet
- Nutritional Guidelines for Kidney Stone Prevention & Management..15
- Foods to Include and Avoid...17
- The Role of Fluids..20

Breakfast
Cranberry Oatmeal Cookies..22
Almond Butter and Banana Smoothie...................................23
Herb and Cheese Baked Eggs..24
Mango Coconut Smoothie Bowl..25
Protein Pancakes..26
Oat Bran Muffins..27
Pear and Ricotta Cheese Toast..28
Tomato and Avocado Toast..29
Apple Walnut Yogurt...30
Chia Seed Pudding..31
Baked Sweet Potato and Yogurt..32
Savory Oatmeal with Poached Egg......................................33
Whole Wheat Waffles...34
Spinach and Mushroom Scrambled Eggs................................35
Pumpkin Spice Smoothie...36
Melon and Cottage Cheese...37
Quinoa Porridge...38
Turkey and Egg Breakfast Burrito......................................39
Zucchini Bread...40

Peaches and Cream Oatmeal..41
Banana Nut Muffins...42
Vegetable Frittata..43
Ricotta Pancakes...44
Avocado Toast on Whole Grain Bread...45

Lunch
Chicken Caesar Salad..46
Quinoa Tabbouleh..47
Turkey and Avocado Wrap...48
Vegetable Stir-Fry with Tofu..49
Beetroot and Goat Cheese Salad...50
Lentil Soup...51
Grilled Salmon with Asparagus..52
Couscous with Roasted Vegetables..53
Caprese Sandwich..54
Butternut Squash Risotto...55
Mediterranean Chickpea Salad...56
Grilled Chicken with Mango Salsa..57
Baked Cod with Herb Crust..58
Vegetable and Hummus Wraps..59
Rice Noodle Salad with Peanut Dressing..60
Roasted Turkey Breast Sandwich...61
Zucchini Noodle Stir-Fry...62
Beef and Broccoli Stir-Fry..63
Greek Yogurt Chicken Salad...64
Balsamic Glazed Salmon..65
Portobello Mushroom Pizza..66
Sesame Chicken Salad...67
Cauliflower Rice Paella...68
Spaghetti Squash with Marinara Sauce..69
Asian Cabbage Salad...70
Tomato Basil Soup...71

Dinner
Grilled Halibut with Lemon Herb Sauce...72
Roasted Chicken with Root Vegetables..73
Pasta Primavera with Whole Wheat Spaghetti.................................74

Baked Trout with Fennel and Citrus Salad..75
Vegetarian Chili...76
Stir-Fried Beef and Broccoli...77
Lemon Garlic Shrimp with Asparagus..78
Cauliflower Steak with Tahini Sauce..79
Grilled Pork Chops with Apple Slaw...80
Seared Scallops with Cauliflower Puree...81
Baked Tilapia with Lemon Parsley Quinoa..82
Chicken Piccata..83
Vegetable Paella...84
Moroccan Spiced Carrot Soup...85
Cod with Parsley Pesto and Steamed Vegetables..................................86
Turkey Stuffed Bell Peppers...87
Squash and Chickpea Moroccan Stew..88
Herbed Lamb Chops with Spinach Salad...89
Tofu and Vegetable Curry...90
Basil Pesto Pasta with Chicken..91
Roasted Duck with Orange Sauce...92
Minted Pea and Barley Risotto...93
Asian Glazed Salmon...94
Chickpea and Spinach Stew..95
Cauliflower and Turmeric Soup...96
Grilled Shrimp and Polenta..97
Lemon Rosemary Grilled Swordfish...98

Desserts
Zucchini Brownies..99
Caramelized Pear Bread Pudding..100
Key Lime Pie with Almond Crust..101
Balsamic Strawberries with Whipped Cream......................................102
Vanilla Bean Panna Cotta...103
Cherry Sorbet...104
Pineapple Upside Down Cake..105
Coconut Macaroons...106
Orange Flavored Ricotta Cheesecake...107
Fig and Honey Yogurt...108
Raspberry Almond Bars..109
Strawberry Kiwi Fruit Tart...110

Berry Crisp with Oat Topping..111
Carrot and Pineapple Cake..112
Blueberry Vanilla Yogurt Popsicles..113

8-WEEK MEAL PLAN..114

Dear Esteemed Reader

As you set out on your gastronomic adventure to improve kidney health, it's essential to remember that each dish in this cookbook has been crafted with care, blending taste with the principles of a kidney stone-managing diet. However, as unique as our fingerprints, so too are our nutritional needs. What works wonders for one might not suit another perfectly.

We encourage you to view these recipes as a canvas rather than a strict rule book. Feel free to adjust spices, swap ingredients, and alter portions to better fit your dietary requirements and palate. Each body has its own story, with individual chapters on health and nutrition, and listening to yours is key.

Before making significant dietary changes, especially if you are currently experiencing or have a history of kidney stones, consulting with a healthcare provider is crucial. They can provide personalized advice that considers your medical history, current health status, and dietary needs. This step ensures that your food choices support your overall health without unintended consequences.

Please also note that the nutritional information provided alongside each recipe is an estimate and can vary based on specific ingredients and portion sizes. Use these details as a guideline to help manage your dietary intake, but adjust as necessary to align with your specific health goals and the advice of your medical professionals.

Furthermore, If our cookbook has brought joy to your kitchen and table, we'd be thrilled to hear about your experiences in an Amazon review. On the flip side, if you stumble upon any hiccups while exploring our recipes, don't hesitate to get in touch at **kloppkingsley@gmail.com.** We're here to support your cooking journey every step of the way.

Introduction

Welcome to the **Kidney Stone Diet Cookbook for Beginners!** Whether you're grappling with kidney stones for the first time, or you're a seasoned pro looking to refine your dietary approach, this book is designed to be your culinary companion on the road to better health. If you're here, you might be intimately familiar with the sharp discomfort that kidney stones can bring. Perhaps you've been through the weary rounds of treatment and are now looking for a proactive way to ensure they remain a part of your past, not your future. Or maybe you're simply interested in preventive health care for your kidneys. Whatever your reason, the decision to focus on what you eat as a way to manage kidney health is a wise and empowering one.

Diet plays a crucial role in managing and preventing kidney stones. Research suggests that certain foods can promote stone formation, while others can help prevent it. This book is designed to guide you through understanding which foods are which, and how to deliciously integrate the good ones into your daily life. Here, you'll find not just recipes, but a new way to think about food and its impact on your body. Let's start with a simple truth: Changing your diet can feel like steering a ship through uncharted waters, especially if you're not used to cooking or are unfamiliar with the ingredients that are beneficial for kidney health. That's why this cookbook aims to make everything as clear and straightforward as possible. Each recipe is not just a set of instructions, but a bridge to a healthier life, designed to be as enjoyable as it is beneficial.

In these pages, we'll explore a variety of dishes that are tailored to reduce the risk of kidney stone formation. From hearty breakfasts that set the tone for your day, to satisfying dinners that your whole family can enjoy, each recipe is crafted with kidney health in mind. But this book goes beyond recipes. It's a guide to understanding the why behind each dietary choice. Why is a high-calcium meal better than a high-oxalate one? Why should someone with kidney stone risks opt for lemon water? These questions and more are answered, giving you not just the how, but the why.

But let's address an important point: Individuality in diet. It's vital to remember that no single diet is perfect for everyone. Our bodies react differently to different foods, influenced by genetics, lifestyle, and existing health conditions. As you use this cookbook, listen to your body and adjust recipes as needed. Feel free to substitute ingredients and tweak quantities to fit your specific needs. And, of course, consult your healthcare provider to tailor these guidelines even better to your personal health context. Remember, the nutritional information provided with each recipe is approximate. Variations in ingredients, brand choices, and even cooking methods can alter nutritional values. Use these numbers as a guide, but let your own circumstances and advice from your healthcare team be your primary reference.

So, grab your apron and let's dive in! Embrace this opportunity to transform your kitchen into a lab where every meal is an experiment in health and flavor. Let's cook our way to fewer kidney stones, better health, and a more vibrant life. Here's to meals that are as nourishing as they are delicious—welcome to your new, stone-free life journey!

Chapter 1: Understanding Kidney Stones

What are Kidney Stones

Kidney stones are hard mineral and salt deposits that form inside the kidneys. They can affect any part of the urinary tract — from the kidneys to the bladder. Often, stones form when the urine becomes concentrated, allowing minerals to crystallize and stick together.

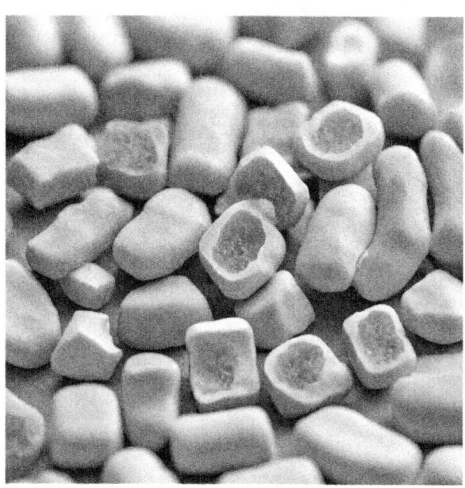

Types of Kidney Stones

Kidney stones are crystalline formations that develop in the urinary tract from dissolved minerals. The types of kidney stones vary based on their chemical composition, which also influences their treatment and prevention strategies.

1. Calcium Stones
Calcium stones are the most prevalent type of kidney stones, typically comprising calcium oxalate and, less commonly, calcium phosphate. Factors influencing their formation include:
- **Oxalate:** Found in many foods (e.g., spinach, rhubarb, nuts), oxalate levels can also be elevated due to high vitamin C intake, metabolic disorders, or intestinal bypass surgery.
- **Phosphate:** High urinary pH can lead to calcium phosphate stone formation, often linked to metabolic conditions like renal tubular acidosis or the use of certain medications such as topiramate.

Prevention generally involves hydration, dietary modifications to reduce oxalate and excessive protein intake, and in some cases, medications that control the amount of calcium or oxalate in the urine.

2. Uric Acid Stones
These stones form when the urine is persistently acidic. A diet rich in purines—substances found in animal proteins such as meats, fish, and shellfish—can increase uric acid in urine. People with gout or undergoing chemotherapy are at higher risk due to elevated uric acid levels.

Prevention and treatment may involve alkalinizing the urine with potassium citrate, reducing dietary purines, and maintaining good hydration to dilute the urine and discourage uric acid stone formation.

3. Struvite Stones

Struvite stones are triggered by infections in the urinary system. They can grow quickly and become quite large, sometimes with little warning. These stones are more common in women because they are more often affected by urinary tract infections.

Managing struvite stones involves treating the underlying infection with antibiotics, and in many cases, removing the stone(s) through surgical procedures. Preventive strategies focus on managing urinary infections and regular monitoring for recurrent stone formation.

4. Cystine Stones

Less common are cystine stones, stemming from a hereditary disorder called cystinuria, characterized by high levels of the amino acid cystine in the urine. Cystine stones can form both in childhood and adulthood.

Treatment typically involves making the urine less acidic, increasing fluid intake to dilute the urine, and medication that binds with cystine to make it less likely to form stones. In severe cases, more complex medical or surgical treatments may be necessary.

Prevention and Management

Prevention strategies for kidney stones generally involve lifestyle and dietary changes. Hydration is crucial; drinking enough water helps dilute the substances in urine that lead to stones. Dietary measures include reducing intake of salt and animal proteins, as well as eating enough dietary calcium to reduce the intestinal absorption of oxalate.

Certain medications can also help manage the risk of recurrence, depending on the stone's type. These might include diuretics or phosphate binders for calcium stones, allopurinol for uric acid stones, antibiotics for struvite stones, or chelating agents for cystine stones.

Causes and Risk Factors

Causes of Kidney Stones
1. **Supersaturation of Urine**: This is the primary physical process leading to stone formation, occurring when waste products form crystals. These include calcium, oxalate, urate, cystine, xanthine, and phosphate. The crystals can grow into larger masses (stones), which can become problematic if they block the urinary tract.
2. **pH Levels**: The acidity or alkalinity of urine can significantly affect the development of certain types of kidney stones. For example, a high pH can lead to the formation of calcium phosphate stones, while a low pH can result in uric acid stones.
3. **Urinary Stasis**: Any condition that blocks the flow of urine will increase the risk of stone formation. Conditions such as kidney cysts, enlarged prostate, or certain types of cancers can contribute to this risk.

Risk Factors
Dietary Factors:
- **High Oxalate Intake**: Foods high in oxalate (e.g., spinach, rhubarb, nuts) can contribute to the formation of calcium oxalate stones if consumed in large amounts.
- **High Sodium Intake**: A diet high in salt increases calcium in the urine, which can lead to the formation of kidney stones.
- **High Protein Intake**: Diets rich in animal protein increase the acid load to the kidneys, increasing the risk of both uric acid and calcium stones.
- **Low Fluid Intake**: Insufficient water intake leads to more concentrated urine, which is more likely to form stones.

Medical Conditions:
- **Hypercalciuria**: This is an inherited condition where the kidneys excrete too much calcium. It is one of the most significant risk factors for calcium stones.
- **Hyperoxaluria**: Excessive oxalate in the urine can occur due to dietary choices, certain intestinal diseases, or inherited disorders.
- **Hyperuricosuria**: This is characterized by too much uric acid in the urine. It can be due to eating too much protein or genetic factors.
- **Cystinuria**: A hereditary condition that results in too much cystine in the urine, leading to the formation of cystine stones.
- **Gout**: Increases uric acid production, leading to the formation of uric acid stones.
- **Urinary tract infections (UTIs)**: These can lead to the formation of struvite stones, especially in women.

Genetic Factors:
Some kidney stones are linked to hereditary factors, making them more likely in certain families, especially in cases of hypercalciuria and cystinuria.

Environmental Factors:
- **Climate**: Hot and dry climates tend to increase the risk of kidney stones due to more fluid loss through sweat, leading to less urine production and higher concentration of stone-forming minerals in the urine.
- **Water Intake**: Regions with a high mineral content in water can have higher incidences of stone formation.

Lifestyle Factors:
- **Obesity**: High body mass index (BMI), large waist size, and weight gain have been linked to an increased risk of kidney stones.
- **Sedentary Lifestyle**: Lack of physical activity is associated with increased risk of stone formation.
- **Certain Medications**: Diuretics (water pills) and calcium-based antacids may increase the risk of forming kidney stones by altering the balance of water, salt, and minerals in urine.

Symptoms
While kidney stones are forming, they typically do not cause any symptoms. However, when they begin to move into the ureter, symptoms can occur suddenly and include severe pain in the side and back, below the ribs, pain that radiates to the lower abdomen and groin, pain during urination, pink, red or brown urine, nausea, and vomiting.

Chapter 2: Basics of the Kidney Stone Diet

Nutritional Guidelines for Kidney Stone Prevention & Management

General Dietary Recommendations
1. **Adequate Fluid Intake:**
   - **Goal**: Aim for 2.5 to 3 liters of total fluid intake per day to produce at least 2.5 liters of urine daily. This dilutes the urine, reducing the risk of stone-forming substances becoming too concentrated.
   - **Types of Fluids**: Water is the best choice. Lemonade and orange juice are beneficial due to their high citric acid content, which can prevent stone formation.
2. **Moderate Calcium Intake:**
   - **Goal**: Consume 1000 to 1200 mg of calcium daily, ideally through dietary sources rather than supplements, which can increase the risk of stone formation if taken without food.
   - **Sources**: Include dairy products like milk, cheese, and yogurt, which are preferred over supplements.
3. **Reduced Sodium Intake:**
   - **Goal**: Limit sodium intake to less than 2300 mg per day. Lower sodium levels in the diet reduce urinary calcium excretion.
   - **Methods**: Avoid processed foods, season foods with herbs instead of salt, and read labels to choose products with lower sodium content.
4. **Controlled Protein Intake:**
   - **Goal**: Moderate consumption of animal proteins to reduce the risk of stone formation.
   - **Impact**: Excessive animal protein increases calcium and uric acid excretion and decreases citrate excretion in urine, all of which contribute to stone formation.
   - **Recommendation**: Opt for plant-based proteins where possible, and limit red meat, poultry, and fish.

5. Limited Oxalate-Rich Foods:
- **Goal**: Reduce intake of high-oxalate foods to decrease oxalate levels in urine.
- **High-Oxalate Foods**: Spinach, rhubarb, almonds, and beetroot, among others. Cooking high-oxalate foods can reduce their oxalate content.

Specific Guidelines for Different Types of Stones

Calcium Oxalate Stones:
- Increase fluid intake, moderate calcium consumption, and limit high-oxalate foods.
- Include foods rich in citrate like lemons, limes, and oranges, which can help prevent the formation of these stones.

Uric Acid Stones:
- Alkalize the urine by consuming a diet higher in fruits and vegetables and lower in animal protein and salt.
- Drink plenty of fluids to dilute the urine and prevent uric acid crystals from forming.

Cystine Stones:
- Maintain high fluid intake to dilute the concentration of cystine in the urine.
- Medications might be necessary to reduce cystine levels and should be discussed with a healthcare provider.

Calcium Phosphate Stones:
- Ensure proper calcium intake and control dietary acid load by increasing fruits and vegetables to maintain a balanced urinary pH.
- Reduce sodium and animal protein intake to decrease phosphate levels in urine.

Foods to Include and Avoid

Managing kidney stone risk through diet involves choosing foods that help prevent stone formation and avoiding those that might contribute to it. The specific recommendations can vary depending on the type of kidney stone, but here are general guidelines for foods to include and avoid:

Foods to Include
1. **Fluids**
   - **Water**: The most crucial element in kidney stone prevention. Aim to drink enough to produce clear or nearly clear urine.
   - **Citrus Beverages**: Lemonade and orange juice are beneficial because they contain citrate, which helps prevent stone formation.
2. **Calcium-Rich Foods**
   - **Dairy Products**: Milk, yogurt, and cheese are good sources of calcium, which, contrary to popular belief, help to bind oxalate in the gut and reduce the risk of calcium oxalate stones.
   - **Vegetables**: Broccoli, kale, and Chinese cabbage offer plant-based calcium.
3. **Plant-Based Proteins**
   - **Legumes**: Lentils, chickpeas, and beans not only provide protein but also fiber, which may help to control weight.
   - **Nuts and Seeds**: In moderate amounts, certain nuts and seeds can be part of a healthy diet but watch the portions because of their high calorie and oxalate contents.
4. **Whole Grains**
   - **Brown Rice, Whole Wheat Bread, and Oats**: These are good sources of nutrients and fiber and have a lower impact on urine calcium than refined grains.

5. **Fruits and Vegetables**
   - **High Fiber Fruits**: Apples, pears, and berries can help keep the urinary system healthy.
   - **Vegetables**: Including a variety of colorful vegetables ensures a broad intake of vitamins and minerals. Aim for low-oxalate options like cauliflower, cucumbers, and peas.
6. **Low-Sodium Foods**
   - **Fresh Meats and Fish**: Processed foods are high in sodium; choose fresh cuts of meat and fresh fish.
   - **Homemade Meals**: Cooking at home allows you to control the amount of salt used.

Foods to Avoid or Limit

1. **High-Oxalate Foods** (for calcium oxalate stones)
   - **Spinach, Rhubarb, Beets, and Swiss Chard**: These are particularly high in oxalate.
   - **Nuts**: Particularly almonds and peanuts.
   - **Potatoes**: Especially sweet potatoes.
2. **High-Sodium Foods**
   - **Processed Foods**: Canned soups, frozen dinners, and processed meats like sausage and deli meats are very high in sodium.
   - **Snack Foods**: Chips, crackers, and pretzels typically have high sodium content.
3. **Animal Proteins**
   - **Red Meat, Poultry, Pork, and Eggs**: High consumption of animal protein can increase the risk of kidney stones and should be consumed in moderation.
   - **Seafood**: Some types like shellfish and anchovies are high in purines, which can increase uric acid in urine.
4. **Sugary Foods and Drinks**
   - **Sodas, Sweetened Beverages**: These can lead to weight gain and increase stone risk.
   - **Candy and Desserts**: High in sugar, contributing to obesity, another risk factor for kidney stones.
5. **Alcohol**
   - While moderate consumption might not directly contribute to stone formation, excessive alcohol intake can lead to dehydration, a significant risk factor for kidney stone development.

Personalized Diet Considerations

Depending on the type of kidney stone one is prone to, the dietary restrictions can vary:

- Those prone to **uric acid stones** may need to limit purine-rich foods like red meat and shellfish.
- For **cystine stones**, maintaining an even higher fluid intake and monitoring specific amino acid intakes might be necessary.
- Those with **calcium phosphate stones** should focus on balancing urinary pH by incorporating more fruits and vegetables and limiting foods that increase urinary calcium (like salt and animal proteins).

The Role of Fluids

Fluid intake plays a crucial role in both the prevention and management of kidney stones. Ensuring adequate hydration is perhaps the most straightforward and effective strategy for reducing the risk of stone formation.

Importance of Hydration
Hydration is key in preventing kidney stones because it dilutes the substances in urine that lead to stones. The more you drink, the more you dilute these substances, which decreases the likelihood that they will crystallize and form stones. Here's how fluids affect various factors related to kidney stones:

1. **Dilution of Urinary Constituents**
The primary mechanism by which fluids prevent stones is by increasing urine volume, which dilutes the concentration of minerals and salts. This reduces the chance that calcium, oxalate, and uric acid will come together to form stones.

2. **Reduction in Urine Supersaturation**
Increased fluid intake decreases the supersaturation of solutes like calcium oxalate and uric acid, which are the most common substances found in kidney stones. Less supersaturated urine is less likely to precipitate crystals.

3. **Increases Urine pH**
Some fluids can alter the pH of urine, which can be instrumental in preventing certain types of stones. For example, a more alkaline (higher pH) urine can help prevent uric acid stones, as uric acid is more soluble in alkaline conditions.

Types of Fluids and Their Specific Roles
While water is universally recommended, other fluids can also play specific roles in kidney stone prevention:
Water
- Simply put, water is the best option for preventing kidney stones. Drinking enough to pass 2.5 to 3 liters of urine per day is a commonly recommended goal.

Citrus Beverages (Lemonade and Orange Juice)
- These contain citrate, a natural inhibitor of kidney stone formation. Citrate binds with calcium in the urine, thereby preventing the formation of calcium oxalate and calcium phosphate stones. Lemonade and other citrus juices should be consumed with no added sugar to maximize benefits.

Coffee and Tea
- Both caffeinated and decaffeinated coffee have been shown to reduce the risk of certain types of kidney stones due to their diuretic effect and content of phytochemicals. Tea, particularly green tea, also offers similar benefits, although black tea might be high in oxalate, which could contribute to calcium oxalate stones if consumed in large amounts.

Alcohol in Moderation
- Moderate consumption of alcohol, particularly wine, has been linked to a reduced risk of kidney stone formation. However, excessive alcohol use can lead to dehydration, counteracting these benefits.

Soft Drinks
- Carbonated beverages, especially those with phosphate additives, are associated with an increased risk of kidney stone formation. However, citrus-flavored sodas might have a lesser risk compared to colas because of their citric acid content.

Recommended Daily Fluid Intake
The general guideline for kidney stone prevention is to drink enough fluids to produce at least 2.5 liters of urine each day. This typically translates to consuming about 3 liters of fluid per day, though individual needs can vary based on factors like climate, body size, and activity level.

Monitoring Hydration
The color of one's urine is a practical way to monitor hydration status; pale yellow to clear urine generally indicates proper hydration, whereas darker urine suggests dehydration. Regular check-ups that include urine tests can also help evaluate how well one is managing fluid intake and modifying the risk of stone formation.

Breakfast

1. **Cranberry Oatmeal Cookies**

Ingredients:
- 1 cup whole wheat flour
- 1/2 teaspoon baking soda
- 1/4 teaspoon salt
- 1/2 cup unsalted butter, softened
- 1/4 cup sugar
- 1/4 cup packed brown sugar
- 1 large egg
- 1 teaspoon vanilla extract
- 1 and 1/2 cups rolled oats
- 1/2 cup dried cranberries

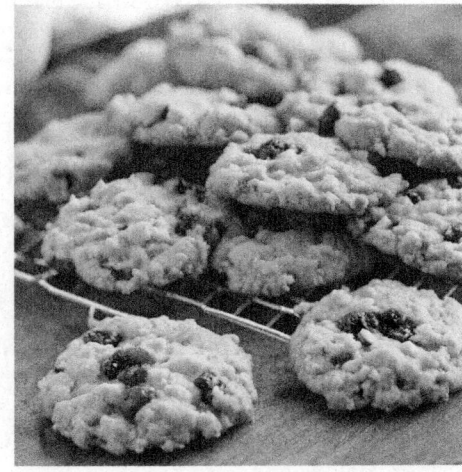

Instructions:
1. Preheat your oven to 350°F (175°C).
2. In a small bowl, mix together the flour, baking soda, and salt.
3. In a larger bowl, cream together the butter, sugar, and brown sugar until smooth.
4. Beat in the egg and vanilla.
5. Gradually blend in the dry ingredients, then stir in the oats and cranberries.
6. Drop by tablespoonfuls onto ungreased cookie sheets.
7. Bake for about 12 minutes, or until the edges are golden.
8. Allow to cool on the baking sheet for a few minutes before transferring to a wire rack to cool completely.

Nutritional Information (per serving):
- Calories: 130
- Protein: 2 g
- Carbohydrates: 18 g
- Fat: 6 g
- Sodium: 55 mg
- Fiber: 2 g

Number of Servings: 24 cookies
Cooking Time: 12 minutes

2. Almond Butter and Banana Smoothie

Ingredients:
- 1 large banana
- 2 tablespoons almond butter
- 1 cup unsweetened almond milk
- 1/2 teaspoon vanilla extract
- 1 cup ice cubes

Instructions:
1. Place the banana, almond butter, almond milk, vanilla extract, and ice cubes in a blender.
2. Blend on high until smooth and creamy.
3. Serve immediately.

Nutritional Information (per serving):
- Calories: 280
- Protein: 5 g
- Carbohydrates: 30 g
- Fat: 16 g
- Sodium: 100 mg
- Fiber: 4 g

Number of Servings: 2
Cooking Time: 5 minutes

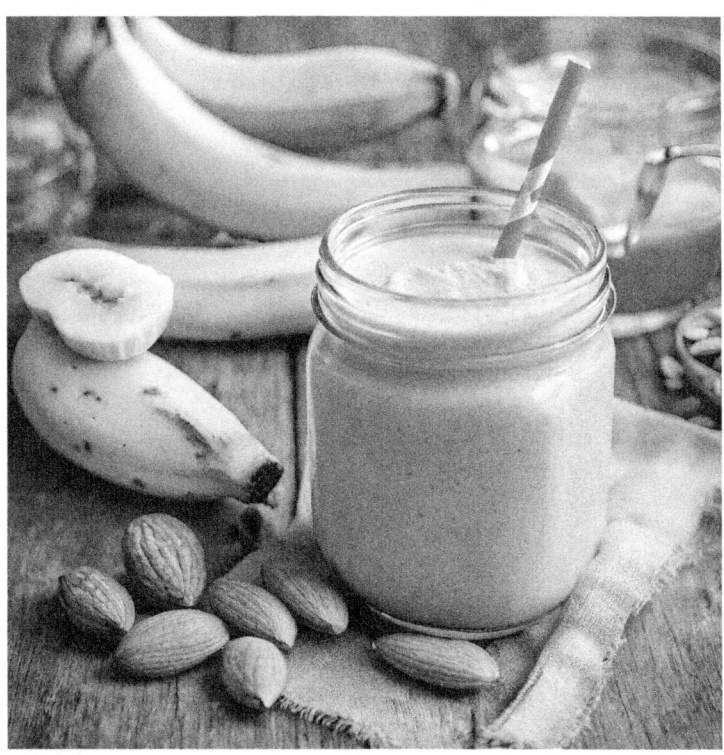

3. Herb and Cheese Baked Eggs

Ingredients:
- 4 large eggs
- 1/4 cup low-fat milk
- 1/2 cup shredded cheddar cheese (low sodium)
- 1 tablespoon chopped fresh parsley
- 1 tablespoon chopped fresh chives
- Salt and pepper to taste (optional and minimal)
- Butter for greasing

Instructions:
1. Preheat your oven to 375°F (190°C).
2. Grease four small ramekins with butter.
3. Crack an egg into each ramekin.
4. Drizzle each egg with a tablespoon of milk.
5. Sprinkle evenly with cheese, parsley, and chives.
6. Season with a pinch of salt and pepper, if using.
7. Place ramekins in a baking dish and pour hot water into the dish to halfway up the sides of the ramekins.
8. Bake for 15-20 minutes, or until the eggs are set to your liking.
9. Carefully remove from the oven and serve hot.

Nutritional Information (per serving):
- Calories: 180
- Protein: 12 g
- Carbohydrates: 2 g
- Fat: 14 g
- Sodium: 170 mg
- Fiber: 0 g

Number of Servings: 4
Cooking Time: 20 minutes

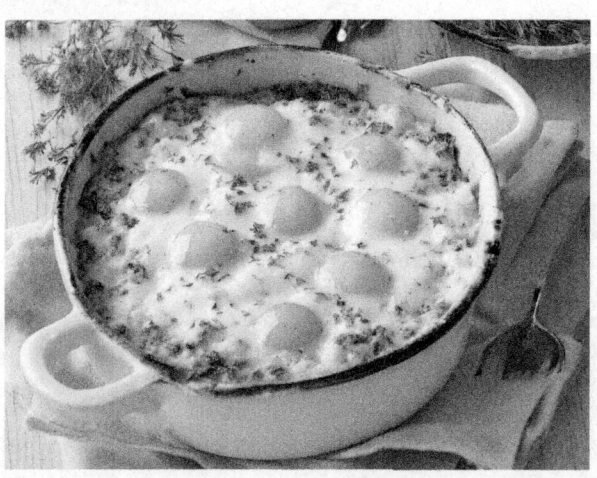

4. Mango Coconut Smoothie Bowl

Ingredients:
- 1 cup frozen mango chunks
- 1/2 cup coconut milk
- 1/2 banana
- 1 tablespoon honey
- Toppings: sliced kiwi, shredded coconut, sliced almonds

Instructions:
1. Blend mango chunks, coconut milk, banana, and honey in a blender until smooth.
2. Pour into a bowl and top with sliced kiwi, shredded coconut, and sliced almonds.
3. Serve immediately.

Nutritional Information (per serving):
- Calories: 300
- Protein: 3 g
- Carbohydrates: 45 g
- Fat: 14 g
- Fiber: 5 g

Number of Servings: 2
Cooking Time: 5 minutes

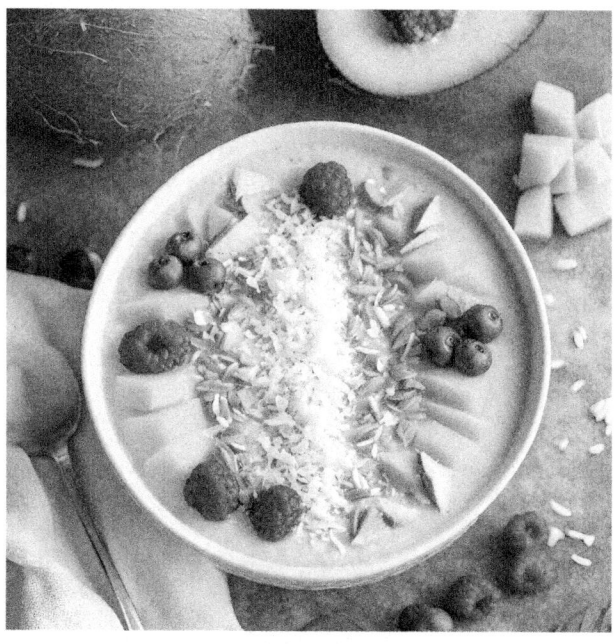

5. Protein Pancakes

Ingredients:
- 1 cup oat flour
- 1/2 cup vanilla whey protein powder
- 1 teaspoon baking powder
- 1/2 teaspoon baking soda
- 1 cup almond milk
- 1 large egg
- 1 tablespoon maple syrup
- 1/2 teaspoon vanilla extract
- Cooking spray

Instructions:
1. Mix oat flour, protein powder, baking powder, and baking soda in a bowl.
2. In another bowl, whisk together almond milk, egg, maple syrup, and vanilla extract.
3. Combine wet and dry ingredients until smooth.
4. Heat a non-stick skillet over medium heat and coat with cooking spray.
5. Pour 1/4 cup of batter for each pancake, cook until bubbles form on the surface, then flip and cook until golden.
6. Serve with additional maple syrup or fresh fruit.

Nutritional Information (per serving):
- Calories: 220
- Protein: 15 g
- Carbohydrates: 30 g
- Fat: 5 g
- Fiber: 4 g

Number of Servings: 4
Cooking Time: 15 minutes

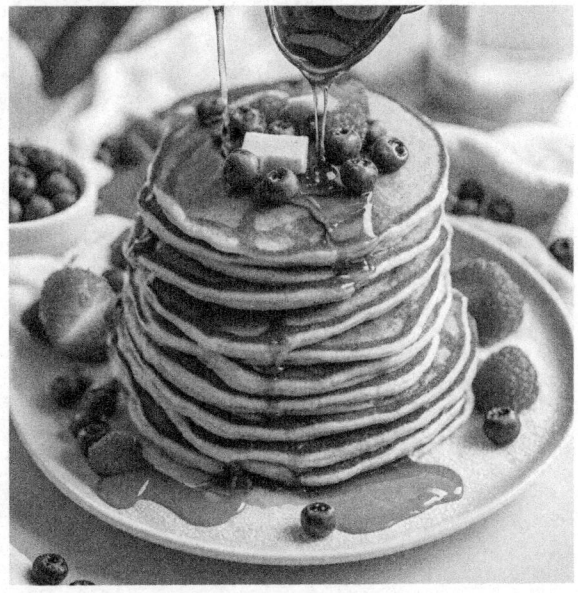

6. Oat Bran Muffins

Ingredients:
- 1 and 1/2 cups oat bran
- 1 cup whole wheat flour
- 1/2 cup brown sugar
- 2 teaspoons baking powder
- 1 teaspoon cinnamon
- 1/2 teaspoon salt
- 1 cup low-fat milk
- 2 large eggs
- 1/4 cup unsweetened applesauce
- 1/4 cup honey
- 1/2 cup raisins (optional)

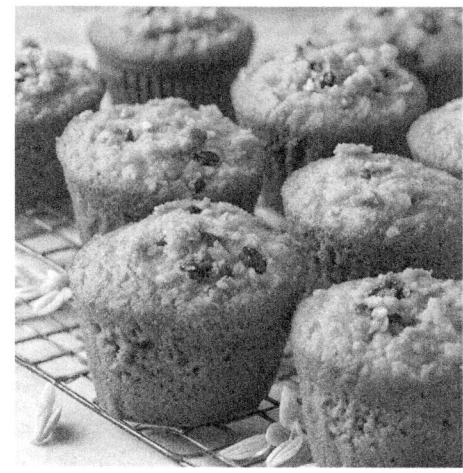

Instructions:
1. Preheat the oven to 375°F (190°C) and line a muffin tin with paper liners.
2. In a large bowl, mix oat bran, flour, brown sugar, baking powder, cinnamon, and salt.
3. In another bowl, whisk together milk, eggs, applesauce, and honey.
4. Combine wet and dry ingredients, then fold in raisins if using.
5. Divide batter among muffin cups and bake for 15-20 minutes or until a toothpick comes out clean.
6. Let cool in the pan for 5 minutes, then transfer to a wire rack to cool completely.

Nutritional Information (per serving):
- Calories: 160
- Protein: 4 g
- Carbohydrates: 28 g
- Fat: 3 g
- Fiber: 4 g

Number of Servings: 12
Cooking Time: 20 minutes

7. Pear and Ricotta Cheese Toast

Ingredients:
- 4 slices whole grain bread
- 1 cup ricotta cheese
- 1 pear, thinly sliced
- 1 tablespoon honey
- A pinch of cinnamon

Instructions:
1. Toast the bread slices to your preference.
2. Spread each slice evenly with ricotta cheese.
3. Top with sliced pear, drizzle with honey, and sprinkle with cinnamon.
4. Serve immediately.

Nutritional Information (per serving):
- Calories: 250
- Protein: 10 g
- Carbohydrates: 35 g
- Fat: 9 g
- Fiber: 5 g

Number of Servings: 4
Cooking Time: 5 minutes

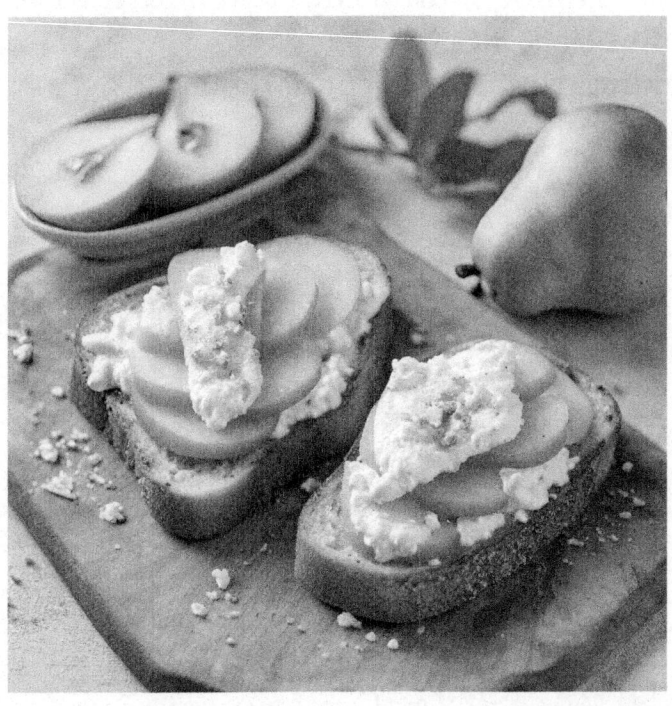

8. Tomato and Avocado Toast

Ingredients:
- 4 slices of whole grain bread
- 1 ripe avocado
- 1 large tomato, sliced
- Salt and pepper to taste
- Drizzle of olive oil (optional)
- Fresh basil leaves (optional)

Instructions:
1. Toast the bread slices until they are golden and crispy.
2. Peel and mash the avocado in a bowl, seasoning lightly with salt and pepper.
3. Spread the mashed avocado evenly over the toasted bread slices.
4. Top each slice with tomato slices, a drizzle of olive oil, and a few basil leaves if using.
5. Season with additional salt and pepper to taste, and serve immediately.

Nutritional Information (per serving):
- Calories: 230
- Protein: 6 g
- Carbohydrates: 27 g
- Fat: 12 g
- Fiber: 7 g

Number of Servings: 4
Cooking Time: 10 minutes

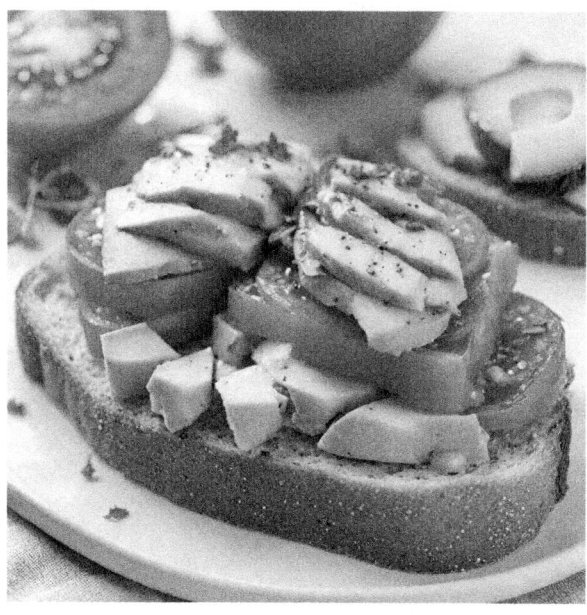

9. Apple Walnut Yogurt

Ingredients:
- 1 cup plain Greek yogurt
- 1 medium apple, chopped
- 1/4 cup walnuts, chopped
- 1 tablespoon honey
- 1/2 teaspoon cinnamon

Instructions:
1. In a bowl, mix the Greek yogurt with chopped apple and walnuts.
2. Drizzle honey over the mixture and sprinkle with cinnamon.
3. Stir everything together until well combined.
4. Serve chilled.

Nutritional Information (per serving):
- Calories: 200
- Protein: 10 g
- Carbohydrates: 18 g
- Fat: 10 g
- Fiber: 3 g

Number of Servings: 2
Cooking Time: 5 minutes (preparation time)

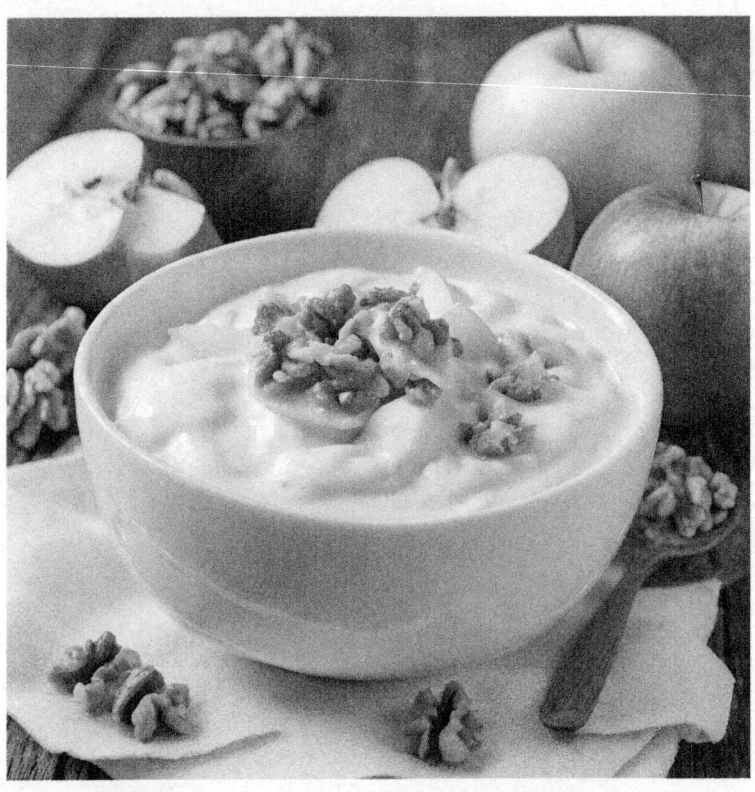

10. Chia Seed Pudding
Ingredients:
- 1/4 cup chia seeds
- 1 cup almond milk
- 1 tablespoon maple syrup
- 1/2 teaspoon vanilla extract
- Fresh berries for topping

Instructions:
1. In a bowl, mix the chia seeds, almond milk, maple syrup, and vanilla extract.
2. Stir well to combine and then let the mixture sit for 5 minutes.
3. Stir again, cover, and refrigerate for at least 2 hours or overnight until it thickens.
4. Serve topped with fresh berries.

Nutritional Information (per serving):
- Calories: 180
- Protein: 4 g
- Carbohydrates: 20 g
- Fat: 9 g
- Fiber: 10 g

Number of Servings: 2

Cooking Time: 2 hours (mostly refrigeration time)

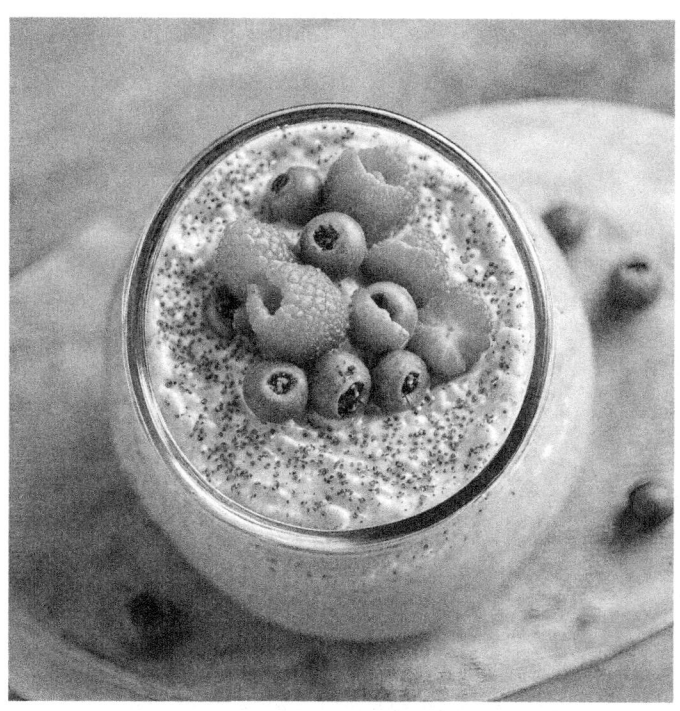

11. Baked Sweet Potato and Yogurt

Ingredients:
- 2 large sweet potatoes
- 1 cup Greek yogurt
- 1 tablespoon honey
- A pinch of cinnamon

Instructions:
1. Preheat the oven to 400°F (200°C).
2. Pierce the sweet potatoes with a fork several times and place them on a baking sheet.
3. Bake for about 45 minutes or until tender.
4. Split the potatoes open and top each with Greek yogurt, a drizzle of honey, and a sprinkle of cinnamon.
5. Serve while warm.

Nutritional Information (per serving):
- Calories: 270
- Protein: 8 g
- Carbohydrates: 50 g
- Fat: 3 g
- Fiber: 7 g

Number of Servings: 2
Cooking Time: 45 minutes

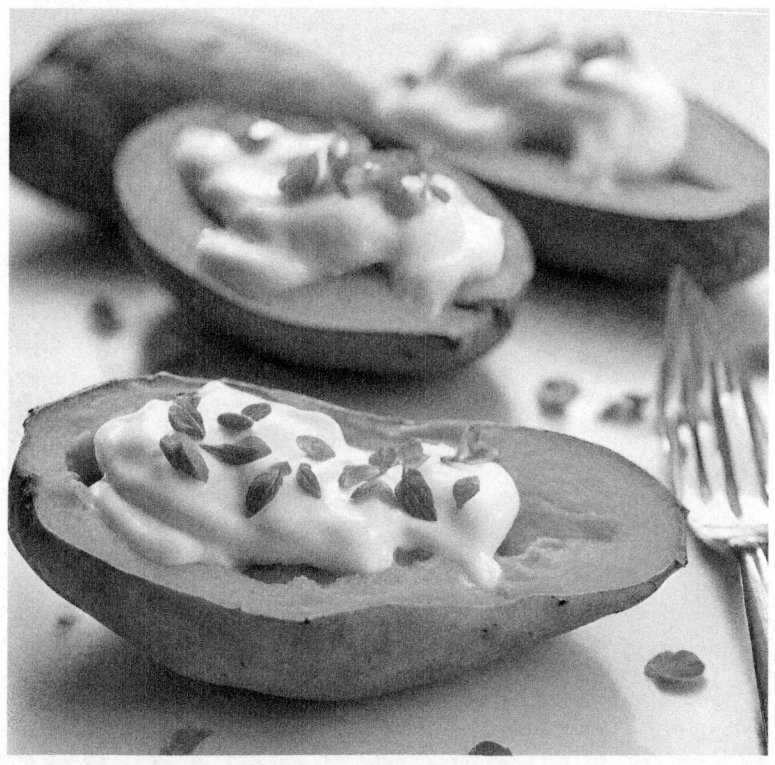

12. Savory Oatmeal with Poached Egg

Ingredients:
- 1 cup rolled oats
- 2 cups water
- Salt and pepper to taste
- 2 eggs
- 1 tablespoon white vinegar
- Chopped scallions and shredded cheese for topping

Instructions:
1. Cook oats with water and a pinch of salt according to package directions until creamy.
2. Meanwhile, bring a small pot of water to a simmer and add vinegar.
3. Crack each egg into a small cup and gently drop into the simmering water.
4. Poach eggs for about 3-4 minutes or until the whites are set but yolks are still runny.
5. Serve the oatmeal in bowls, top each with a poached egg, scallions, shredded cheese, and a sprinkle of pepper.

Nutritional Information (per serving):
- Calories: 300
- Protein: 14 g
- Carbohydrates: 38 g
- Fat: 10 g
- Fiber: 6 g

Number of Servings: 2
Cooking Time: 20 minutes

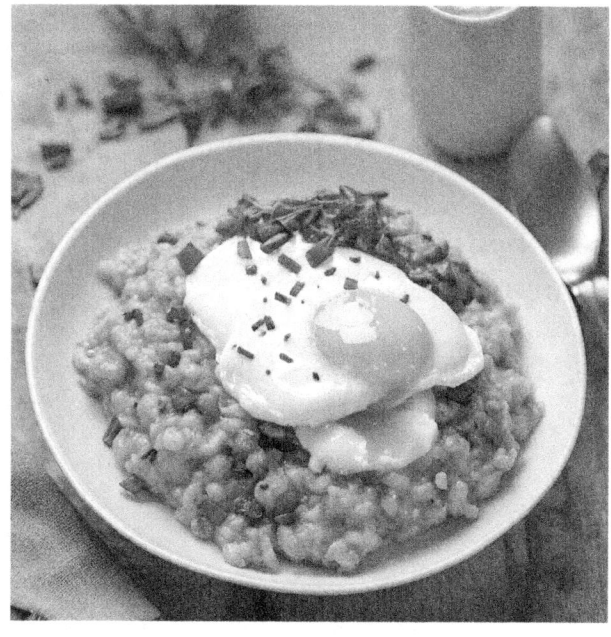

13. Whole Wheat Waffles

Ingredients:
- 2 cups whole wheat flour
- 2 teaspoons baking powder
- 1/2 teaspoon salt
- 2 tablespoons sugar
- 2 eggs
- 1 and 3/4 cups milk
- 1/3 cup vegetable oil
- 1 teaspoon vanilla extract

Instructions:
1. Preheat your waffle iron.
2. In a large bowl, whisk together flour, baking powder, salt, and sugar.
3. In another bowl, beat eggs and then mix with milk, oil, and vanilla extract.
4. Pour the wet ingredients into the dry ingredients and stir until just combined.
5. Cook according to your waffle iron's instructions until golden and crisp.
6. Serve hot with your choice of toppings like fresh fruit or syrup.

Nutritional Information (per serving):
- Calories: 290
- Protein: 8 g
- Carbohydrates: 35 g
- Fat: 14 g
- Fiber: 4 g

Number of Servings: 6
Cooking Time: 15 minutes

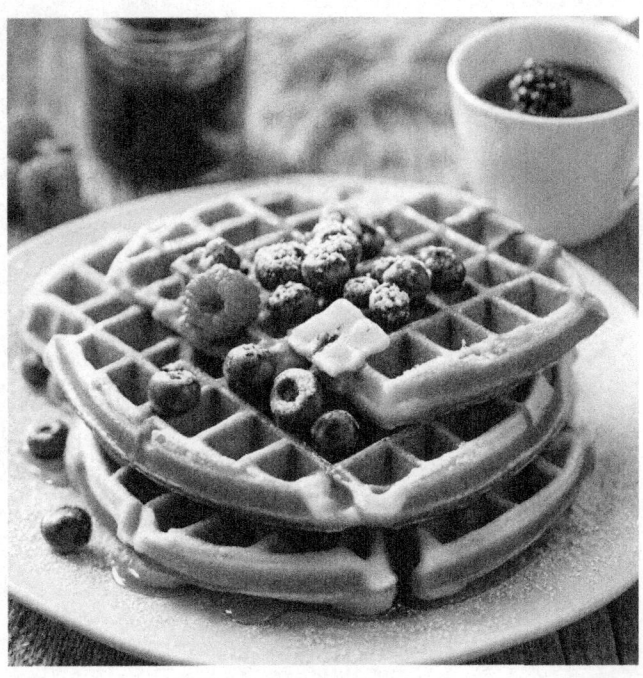

14. Spinach and Mushroom Scrambled Eggs

Ingredients:
- 4 large eggs
- 1 cup fresh spinach, chopped
- 1/2 cup mushrooms, sliced
- 1/4 cup skim milk
- Salt and pepper to taste (minimal salt)
- 1 tablespoon olive oil

Instructions:
1. In a bowl, whisk the eggs and milk together, seasoning lightly with salt and pepper.
2. Heat the olive oil in a non-stick skillet over medium heat.
3. Add the mushrooms and sauté until they are soft, about 5 minutes.
4. Add the spinach and cook until just wilted.
5. Pour the egg mixture into the skillet, and cook, stirring gently until the eggs are set and fluffy.
6. Serve immediately.

Nutritional Information (per serving):
- Calories: 150
- Protein: 10 g
- Carbohydrates: 3 g
- Fat: 11 g
- Fiber: 1 g
- Sodium: 170 mg

Number of Servings: 2
Cooking Time: 15 minutes

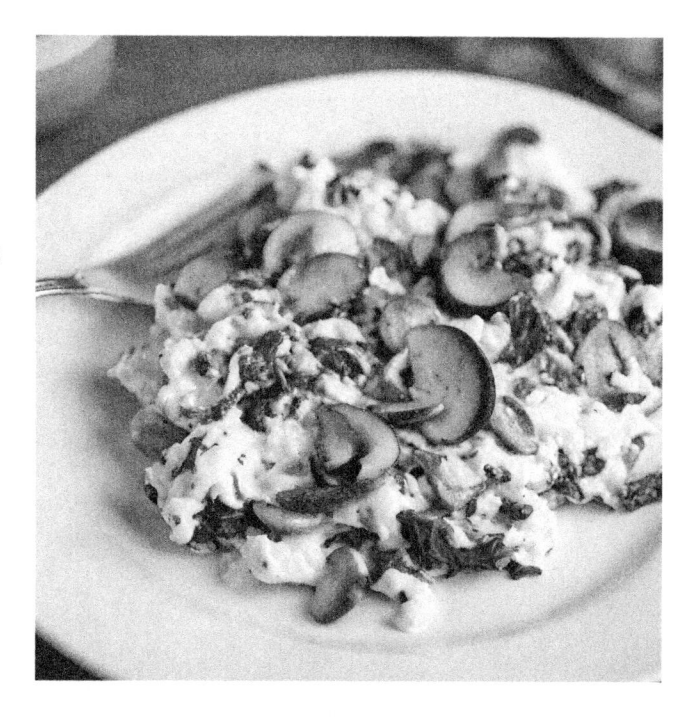

15. Pumpkin Spice Smoothie
Ingredients:
- 1/2 cup pumpkin puree (canned or fresh)
- 1 cup almond milk
- 1 banana
- 1/2 teaspoon pumpkin pie spice
- 1 tablespoon maple syrup
- Ice cubes

Instructions:
1. Place all ingredients in a blender.
2. Blend on high until smooth.
3. Serve chilled, garnished with a sprinkle of pumpkin pie spice if desired.

Nutritional Information (per serving):
- Calories: 200
- Protein: 2 g
- Carbohydrates: 44 g
- Fat: 2.5 g
- Fiber: 5 g
- Sodium: 80 mg

Number of Servings: 2
Cooking Time: 5 minutes

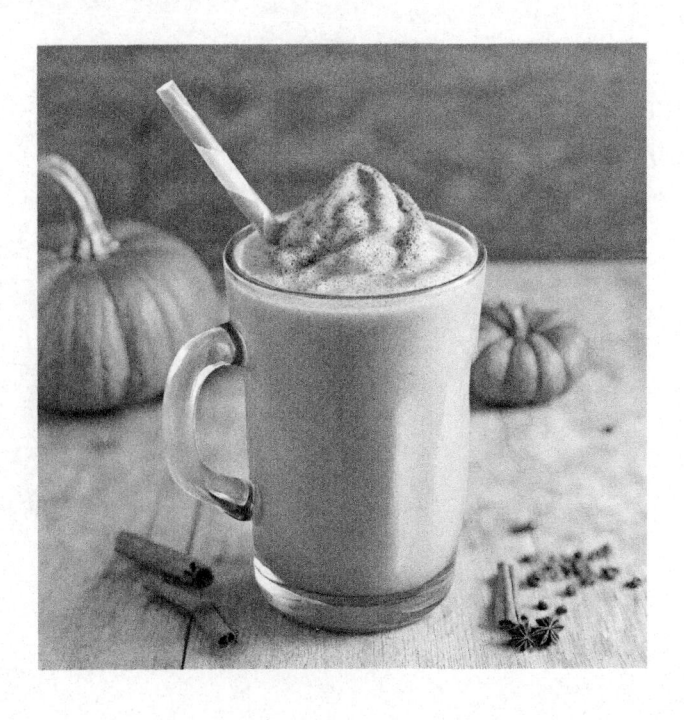

16. Melon and Cottage Cheese

Ingredients:
- 1 cup cantaloupe, cubed
- 1 cup honeydew melon, cubed
- 1 cup low-fat cottage cheese
- Fresh mint for garnish (optional)

Instructions:
1. Arrange the cubed melon on a plate or in a bowl.
2. Top with cottage cheese.
3. Garnish with fresh mint if using.
4. Serve chilled.

Nutritional Information (per serving):
- Calories: 180
- Protein: 14 g
- Carbohydrates: 20 g
- Fat: 4 g
- Fiber: 1 g
- Sodium: 350 mg

Number of Servings: 2

Cooking Time: 5 minutes (preparation time)

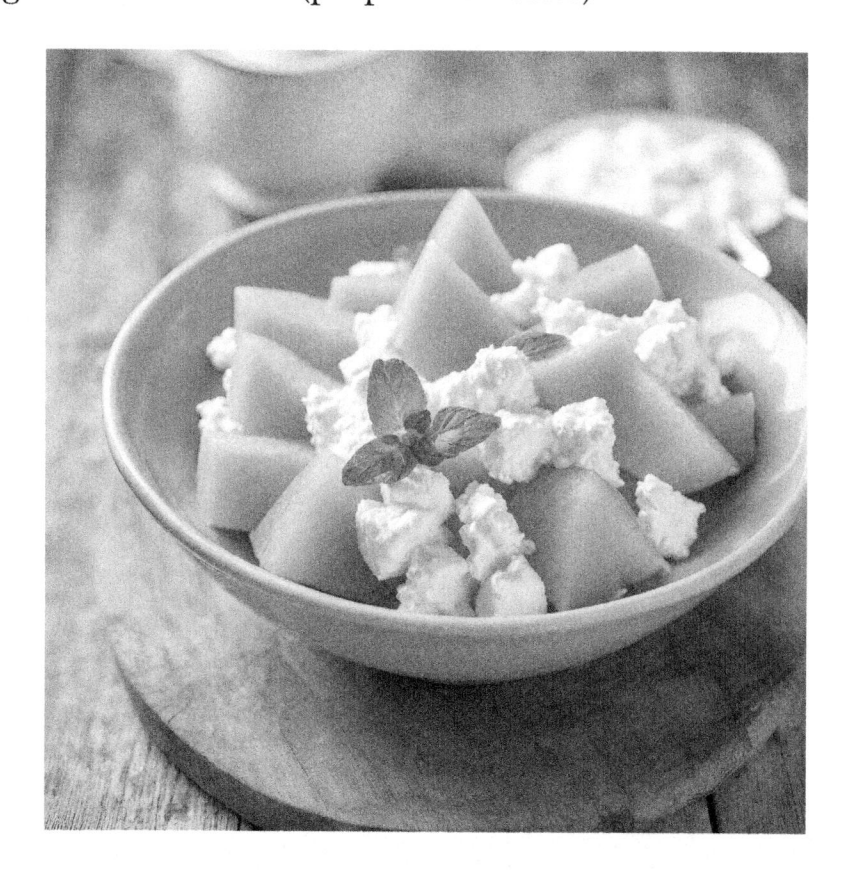

17. Quinoa Porridge

Ingredients:
- 1 cup quinoa, rinsed
- 2 cups water
- 1 cup almond milk
- 1 apple, chopped
- 1 teaspoon cinnamon
- 1 tablespoon honey or maple syrup

Instructions:
1. Combine quinoa and water in a medium saucepan. Bring to a boil.
2. Reduce heat to low and simmer covered for 15 minutes or until quinoa is tender.
3. Stir in almond milk, chopped apple, cinnamon, and sweetener.
4. Cook for an additional 5 minutes, stirring occasionally.
5. Serve warm.

Nutritional Information (per serving):
- Calories: 270
- Protein: 8 g
- Carbohydrates: 50 g
- Fat: 5 g
- Fiber: 6 g
- Sodium: 30 mg

Number of Servings: 2
Cooking Time: 25 minutes

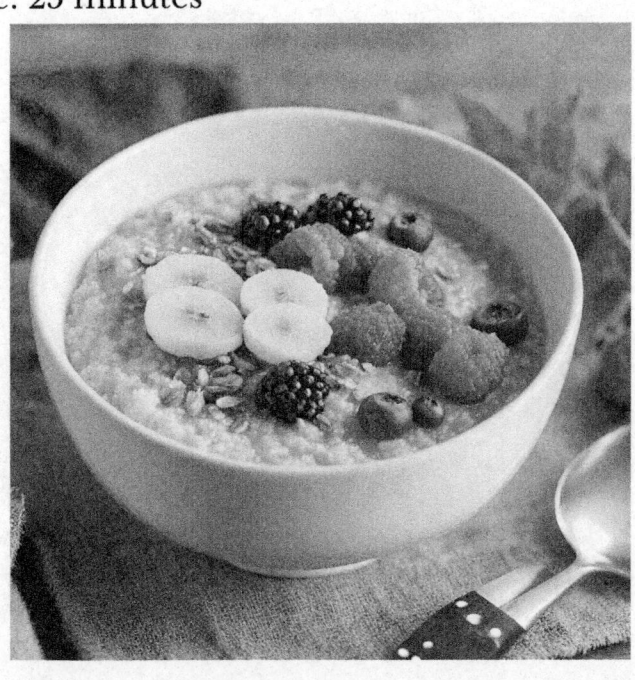

18. Turkey and Egg Breakfast Burrito

Ingredients:
- 2 whole wheat tortillas
- 4 egg whites
- 1/2 cup cooked turkey breast, chopped
- 1/4 cup low-fat cheddar cheese, shredded
- 1/4 cup bell pepper, diced
- 1/4 cup onion, diced
- Salt and pepper to taste (minimal salt)
- Cooking spray

Instructions:
1. Spray a non-stick skillet with cooking spray and heat over medium heat.
2. Sauté bell pepper and onion until soft.
3. Add egg whites and turkey, scrambling until the eggs are cooked through.
4. Warm the tortillas in a microwave or another skillet.
5. Divide the egg mixture among the tortillas, top with cheese, and roll up.
6. Serve immediately.

Nutritional Information (per serving):
- Calories: 250
- Protein: 28 g
- Carbohydrates: 22 g
- Fat: 7 g
- Fiber: 3 g
- Sodium: 400 mg

Number of Servings: 2
Cooking Time: 20 minutes

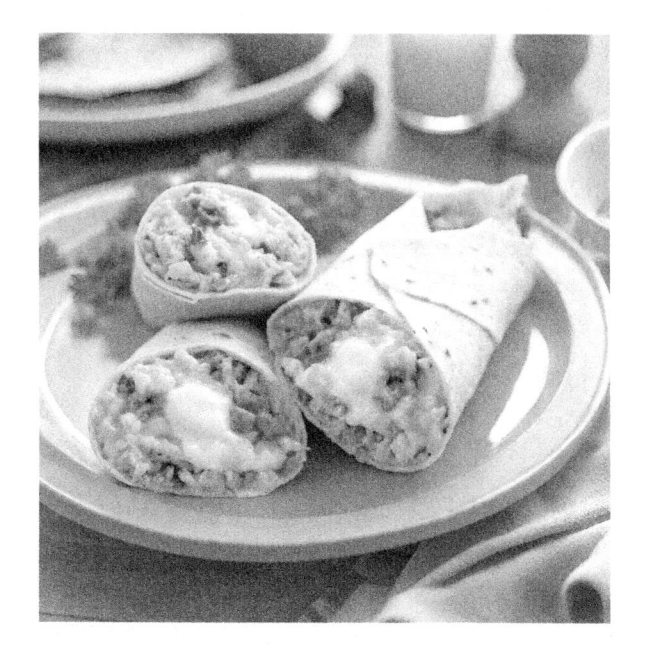

19. Zucchini Bread

Ingredients:
- 1 and 1/2 cups whole wheat flour
- 1/2 teaspoon baking soda
- 1/2 teaspoon baking powder
- 1 teaspoon cinnamon
- 1/4 teaspoon salt
- 1 cup grated zucchini
- 1/2 cup unsweetened applesauce
- 1/2 cup honey
- 2 eggs
- 1/4 cup vegetable oil
- 1 teaspoon vanilla extract

Instructions:
1. Preheat oven to 350°F (175°C). Grease and flour a loaf pan.
2. In a bowl, mix flour, baking soda, baking powder, cinnamon, and salt.
3. In another bowl, combine zucchini, applesauce, honey, eggs, oil, and vanilla.
4. Stir wet ingredients into dry until just moistened.
5. Pour batter into prepared pan.
6. Bake for 50 minutes or until a toothpick inserted into the center comes out clean.
7. Cool in pan on a wire rack before slicing.

Nutritional Information (per serving):
- Calories: 180
- Protein: 3 g
- Carbohydrates: 28 g
- Fat: 7 g
- Fiber: 3 g
- Sodium: 150 mg

Number of Servings: 12
Cooking Time: 50 minutes

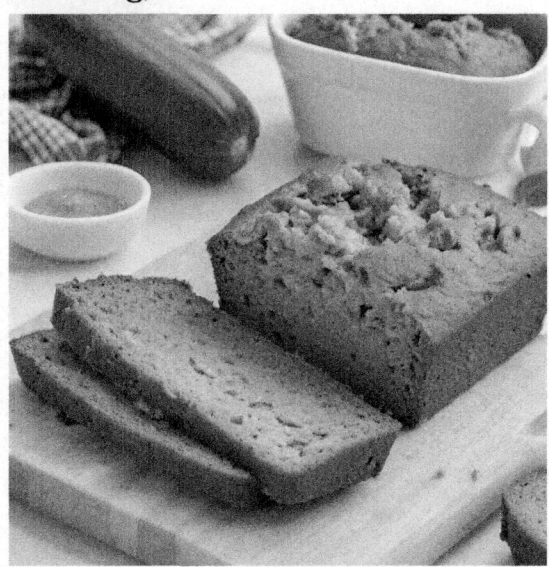

20. Peaches and Cream Oatmeal

Ingredients:
- 1 cup rolled oats
- 2 cups water
- 1 cup sliced fresh peaches
- 1/2 cup almond milk
- 1 tablespoon honey
- 1/4 teaspoon cinnamon

Instructions:
1. Bring water to a boil in a saucepan. Add oats and reduce heat to a simmer.
2. Cook f il oats are soft.
3. Stir in Cook for anothe
4. Serve h

Nutrition
- Calorie
- Protein
- Carboh
- Fat: 4 g
- Fiber:
- Sodium

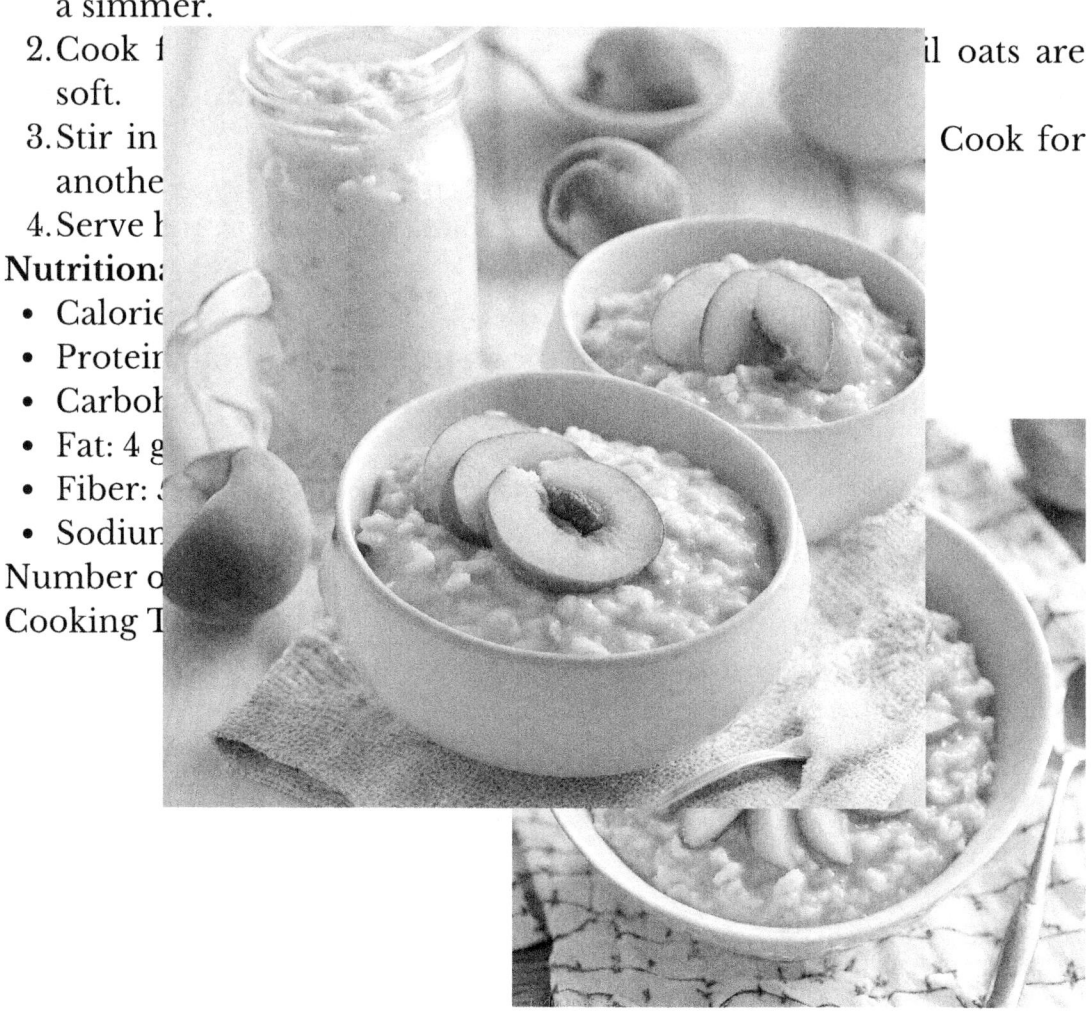

Number o
Cooking T

21. Banana Nut Muffins

Ingredients:
- 1 and 1/2 cups whole wheat flour
- 1 teaspoon baking soda
- 1/4 teaspoon salt
- 3 ripe bananas, mashed
- 1/4 cup honey
- 1 tablespoon vanilla extract
- 1/4 cup unsweetened applesauce
- 1/2 cup chopped walnuts
- 2 eggs

Instructions:
1. Preheat your oven to 350°F (175°C) and line a muffin tin with paper liners or grease with non-stick spray.
2. In a bowl, combine flour, baking soda, and salt.
3. In another bowl, mix mashed bananas, honey, vanilla extract, applesauce, and eggs.
4. Gradually mix the dry ingredients into the wet ingredients, stirring until just combined. Fold in the chopped walnuts.
5. Spoon the batter into the muffin tins, filling each cup about two-thirds full.
6. Bake for 20-25 minutes, or until a toothpick inserted into the center comes out clean.
7. Allow to cool for a few minutes in the pan, then move to a wire rack to cool completely.

Nutritional Information (per serving):
- Calories: 190
- Protein: 4 g
- Carbohydrates: 30 g
- Fat: 7 g
- Fiber: 3 g
- Sodium: 150 mg

Number of Servings: 12
Cooking Time: 25 minutes

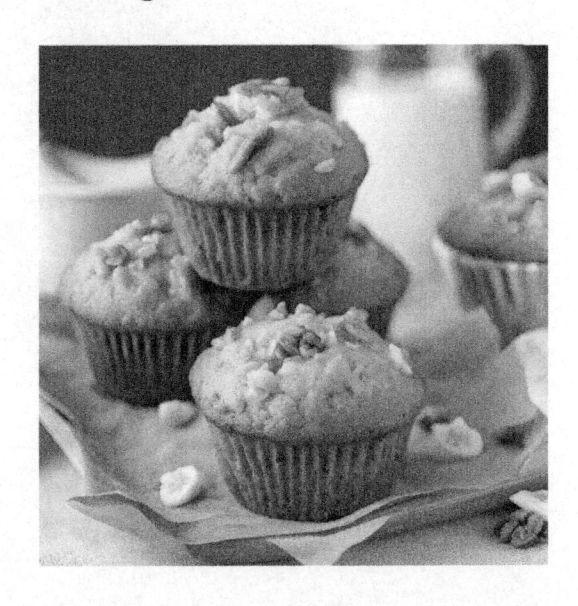

22. Vegetable Frittata

Ingredients:
- 6 large eggs
- 1/2 cup milk
- 1 cup chopped spinach
- 1/2 cup diced tomatoes
- 1/2 cup chopped bell peppers
- 1/4 cup diced onions
- 1/2 teaspoon salt
- 1/4 teaspoon pepper
- 1 tablespoon olive oil

Instructions:
1. Preheat oven to 400°F (200°C).
2. In a bowl, whisk together eggs, milk, salt, and pepper.
3. Heat olive oil in an oven-safe skillet over medium heat.
4. Sauté onions and bell peppers until softened.
5. Add spinach and tomatoes and cook until spinach is wilted.
6. Pour the egg mixture over the vegetables in the skillet.
7. Cook without stirring for about 5 minutes until the edges start to set.
8. Transfer skillet to oven and bake for 10-15 minutes, or until the frittata is set and golden on top.
9. Let cool slightly before cutting into wedges and serving.

Nutritional Information (per serving):
- Calories: 130
- Protein: 9 g
- Carbohydrates: 5 g
- Fat: 9 g
- Fiber: 1 g
- Sodium: 250 mg

Number of Servings: 4

Cooking Time: 25 minutes

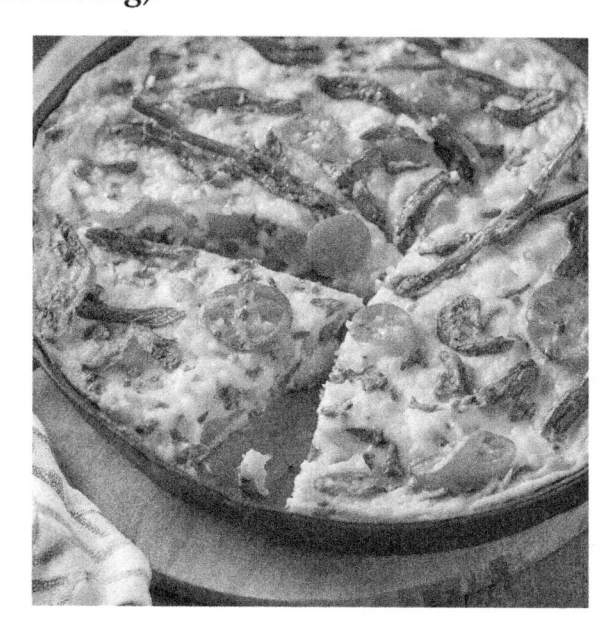

23. Ricotta Pancakes

Ingredients:
- 1 cup whole wheat flour
- 2 teaspoons baking powder
- 1/2 teaspoon salt
- 1 cup ricotta cheese
- 3/4 cup milk
- 2 eggs, separated
- 1 tablespoon sugar
- 1 teaspoon vanilla extract
- Butter or cooking spray for cooking

Instructions:
1. In a bowl, mix together flour, baking powder, and salt.
2. In another bowl, combine ricotta, milk, egg yolks, sugar, and vanilla extract.
3. Stir the ricotta mixture into the flour mixture until just combined.
4. In a separate bowl, beat the egg whites until stiff peaks form, then fold into the batter.
5. Heat a non-stick skillet over medium heat and grease lightly with butter or spray.
6. Pour 1/4 cup of batter for each pancake and cook until bubbles form on the surface, then flip and cook until golden brown.
7. Serve hot with maple syrup or fresh fruit.

Nutritional Information (per serving):
- Calories: 220
- Protein: 11 g
- Carbohydrates: 21 g
- Fat: 10 g
- Fiber: 2 g
- Sodium: 390 mg

Number of Servings: 4
Cooking Time: 15 minutes

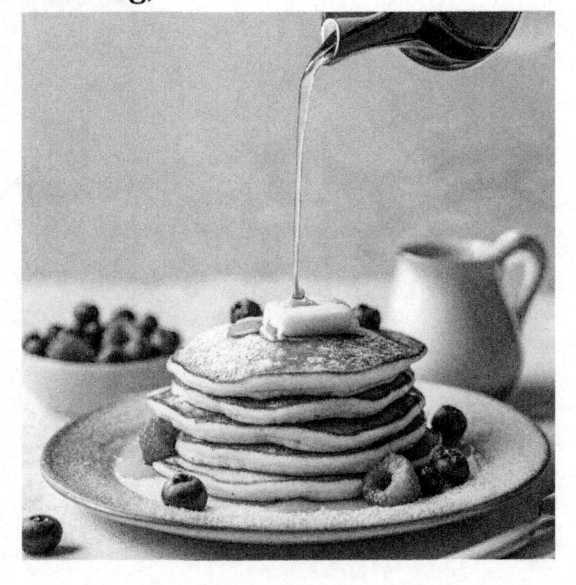

24. Avocado Toast on Whole Grain Bread
Ingredients:
- 4 slices whole grain bread
- 2 ripe avocados
- Juice of 1 lime
- Salt and pepper to taste
- 1/4 cup sliced radishes
- 1/4 cup alfalfa sprouts

Instructions:
1. Toast the bread slices until golden and crisp.
2. In a bowl, mash the avocados with lime juice, salt, and pepper.
3. Spread the mashed avocado evenly over each slice of toasted bread.
4. Top with sliced radishes and alfalfa sprouts.
5. Serve immediately.

Nutritional Information (per serving):
- Calories: 250
- Protein: 6 g
- Carbohydrates: 27 g
- Fat: 14 g
- Fiber: 8 g
- Sodium: 200 mg

Number of Servings: 4
Cooking Time: 10 minutes

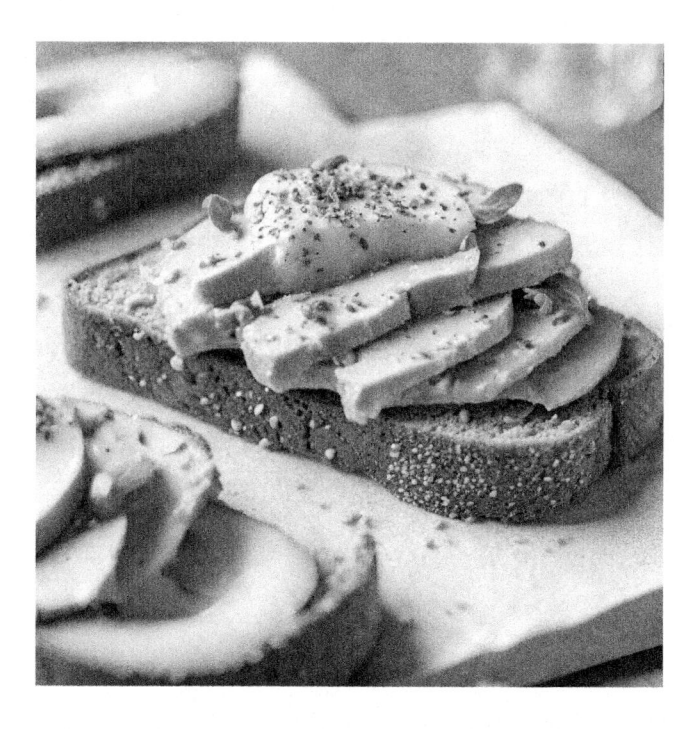

Lunch

1. Chicken Caesar Salad
Ingredients:
- 2 boneless, skinless chicken breasts
- 6 cups chopped Romaine lettuce
- 1/2 cup low-fat Caesar dressing
- 1/4 cup grated Parmesan cheese
- 1 cup whole grain croutons
- Salt and pepper to taste

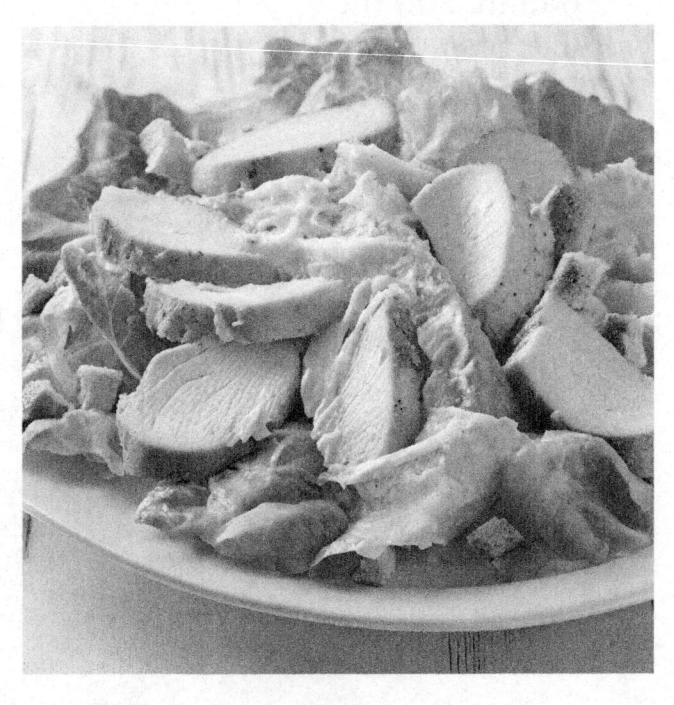

Instructions:
1. Season chicken breasts with salt and pepper.
2. Grill chicken over medium heat until cooked through, about 6-7 minutes per side.
3. Let chicken rest for a few minutes, then slice thinly.
4. Toss Romaine lettuce with Caesar dressing in a large bowl.
5. Top with sliced chicken, croutons, and Parmesan cheese.
6. Serve immediately.

Nutritional Information (per serving):
- Calories: 350
- Protein: 28 g
- Carbohydrates: 18 g
- Fat: 18 g
- Fiber: 3 g
- Sodium: 450 mg

Number of Servings: 4
Cooking Time: 20 minutes

2. Quinoa Tabbouleh
Ingredients:
- 1 cup quinoa, rinsed
- 2 cups water
- 1 cup chopped parsley
- 1/2 cup chopped mint
- 1/2 cup diced cucumber
- 1/2 cup diced tomato
- 1/4 cup lemon juice
- 1/4 cup olive oil
- Salt and pepper to taste

Instructions:
1. Bring water to a boil, add quinoa, reduce to a simmer, cover, and cook until water is absorbed and quinoa is tender, about 15 minutes.
2. Fluff quinoa with a fork and let cool.
3. Once cooled, mix quinoa with parsley, mint, cucumber, and tomato.
4. Dress with lemon juice and olive oil, and season with salt and pepper.
5. Chill in the refrigerator before serving.

Nutritional Information (per serving):
- Calories: 240
- Protein: 6 g
- Carbohydrates: 28 g
- Fat: 12 g
- Fiber: 5 g
- Sodium: 30 mg

Number of Servings: 4
Cooking Time: 25 minutes

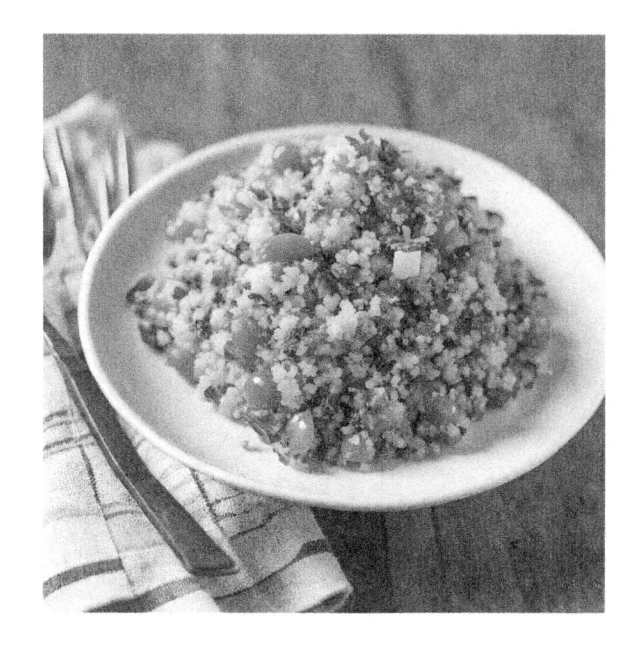

3. Turkey and Avocado Wrap

Ingredients:
- 4 whole wheat tortillas
- 8 ounces sliced turkey breast
- 1 ripe avocado, sliced
- 1 cup shredded lettuce
- 1/2 cup sliced tomatoes
- 2 tablespoons ranch dressing
- Salt and pepper to taste

Instructions:
1. Lay out tortillas on a flat surface.
2. Spread each tortilla with ranch dressing.
3. Layer turkey, avocado slices, lettuce, and tomatoes evenly among the tortillas.
4. Season with a pinch of salt and pepper.
5. Roll up the tortillas tightly, cut in half, and serve.

Nutritional Information (per serving):
- Calories: 320
- Protein: 20 g
- Carbohydrates: 28 g
- Fat: 16 g
- Fiber: 5 g
- Sodium: 560 mg

Number of Servings: 4
Cooking Time: 10 minutes

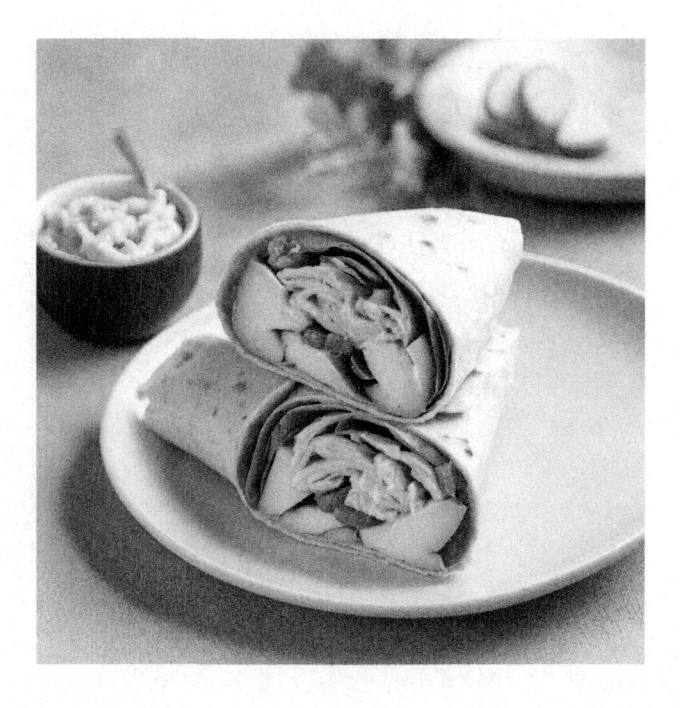

4. Vegetable Stir-Fry with Tofu

Ingredients:
- 1 block firm tofu, drained and cubed
- 2 tablespoons soy sauce (low sodium)
- 1 tablespoon sesame oil
- 1 cup broccoli florets
- 1/2 cup sliced carrots
- 1/2 cup sliced bell peppers
- 1/2 cup snow peas
- 1 tablespoon minced ginger
- 2 cloves garlic, minced
- 1/4 cup water or vegetable broth

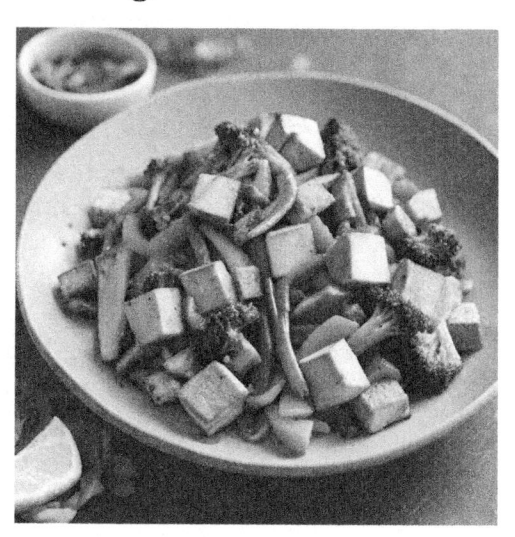

Instructions:
1. Heat sesame oil in a large skillet over medium-high heat.
2. Add tofu and soy sauce, and cook until golden brown on all sides, about 5-7 minutes.
3. Remove tofu and set aside.
4. In the same skillet, add ginger and garlic, and sauté for 30 seconds.
5. Add broccoli, carrots, bell peppers, and snow peas, stir-frying for about 5 minutes.
6. Add water or broth, bring to a simmer, and return the tofu to the skillet.
7. Cook until vegetables are tender and tofu is heated through, about 3 more minutes.
8. Serve hot.

Nutritional Information (per serving):
- Calories: 180
- Protein: 12 g
- Carbohydrates: 10 g
- Fat: 10 g
- Fiber: 3 g
- Sodium: 300 mg

Number of Servings: 4
Cooking Time: 20 minutes

5. Beetroot and Goat Cheese Salad

Ingredients:
- 4 medium beetroots, peeled and diced
- 1 tablespoon olive oil
- Salt and pepper to taste
- 4 cups mixed salad greens
- 1/2 cup crumbled goat cheese
- 1/4 cup walnuts, chopped
- 2 tablespoons balsamic vinegar

Instructions:
1. Preheat the oven to 400°F (200°C).
2. Toss the diced beetroots with olive oil, salt, and pepper.
3. Spread them on a baking sheet and roast for 30-35 minutes, until tender.
4. Allow the beetroots to cool slightly.
5. In a large salad bowl, combine the roasted beetroots, salad greens, goat cheese, and chopped walnuts.
6. Drizzle with balsamic vinegar and toss gently to combine.
7. Serve immediately.

Nutritional Information (per serving):
- Calories: 250
- Protein: 8 g
- Carbohydrates: 18 g
- Fat: 17 g
- Fiber: 5 g
- Sodium: 260 mg

Number of Servings: 4
Cooking Time: 45 minutes

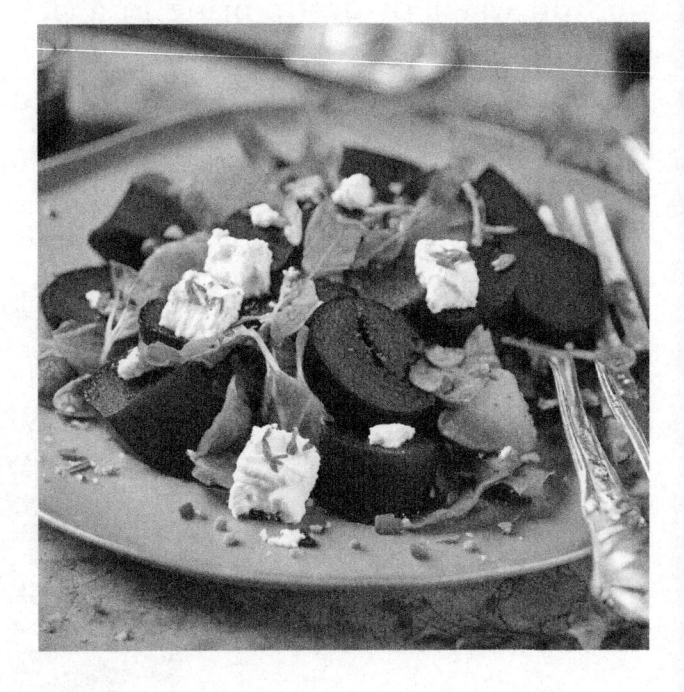

6. Lentil Soup

Ingredients:
- 1 cup dried lentils, rinsed
- 1 tablespoon olive oil
- 1 onion, chopped
- 2 carrots, diced
- 2 celery stalks, diced
- 2 cloves garlic, minced
- 1 teaspoon ground cumin
- 6 cups vegetable broth
- 1 bay leaf
- Salt and pepper to taste
- 2 tablespoons chopped fresh parsley

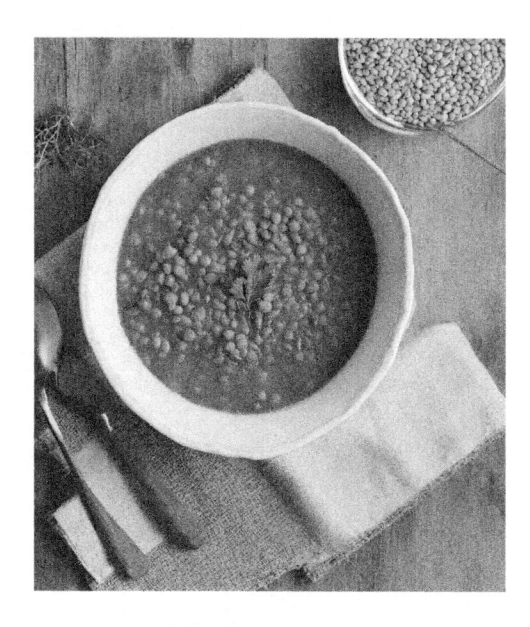

Instructions:
1. Heat olive oil in a large pot over medium heat.
2. Add onion, carrots, celery, and garlic, cooking until the vegetables are softened, about 5 minutes.
3. Stir in cumin and cook for an additional minute.
4. Add lentils, vegetable broth, and bay leaf. Bring to a boil.
5. Reduce heat and simmer, covered, until lentils are tender, about 30 minutes.
6. Season with salt and pepper.
7. Remove the bay leaf and sprinkle with fresh parsley before serving.

Nutritional Information (per serving):
- Calories: 230
- Protein: 14 g
- Carbohydrates: 35 g
- Fat: 4 g
- Fiber: 15 g
- Sodium: 300 mg

Number of Servings: 4
Cooking Time: 45 minutes

7. Grilled Salmon with Asparagus

Ingredients:
- 4 salmon fillets (4 ounces each)
- 1 tablespoon olive oil
- Salt and pepper to taste
- 1 pound asparagus, trimmed
- Lemon wedges, for serving

Instructions:
1. Preheat grill to medium-high heat.
2. Brush salmon and asparagus with olive oil and season with salt and pepper.
3. Grill salmon, skin side down, for 6-8 minutes, then flip and cook for an additional 3-4 minutes, or until cooked through.
4. Grill asparagus alongside salmon for about 4-5 minutes, turning occasionally, until tender and charred.
5. Serve the salmon and asparagus with lemon wedges on the side.

Nutritional Information (per serving):
- Calories: 260
- Protein: 25 g
- Carbohydrates: 5 g
- Fat: 16 g
- Fiber: 2 g
- Sodium: 75 mg

Number of Servings: 4
Cooking Time: 20 minutes

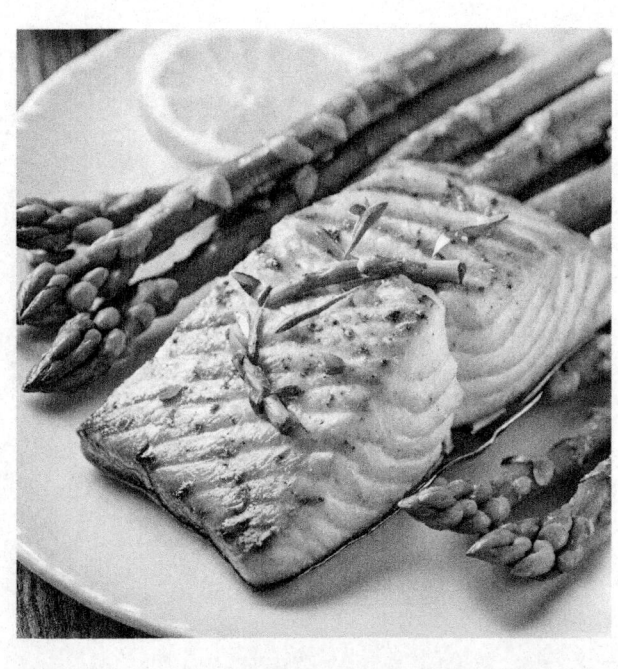

8. Couscous with Roasted Vegetables

Ingredients:
- 1 cup couscous
- 2 cups vegetable broth
- 1 zucchini, diced
- 1 bell pepper, diced
- 1 red onion, diced
- 2 tablespoons olive oil
- Salt and pepper to taste
- 1/4 cup chopped fresh parsley

Instructions:
1. Preheat oven to 425°F (220°C).
2. Toss zucchini, bell pepper, and red onion with olive oil, salt, and pepper.
3. Spread vegetables on a baking sheet and roast for 20 minutes, until tender.
4. Meanwhile, bring vegetable broth to a boil in a medium pot.
5. Stir in couscous, cover, remove from heat, and let sit for 5 minutes.
6. Fluff couscous with a fork and mix in roasted vegetables and fresh parsley.
7. Serve warm.

Nutritional Information (per serving):
- Calories: 250
- Protein: 6 g
- Carbohydrates: 42 g
- Fat: 7 g
- Fiber: 4 g
- Sodium: 300 mg

Number of Servings: 4
Cooking Time: 30 minutes

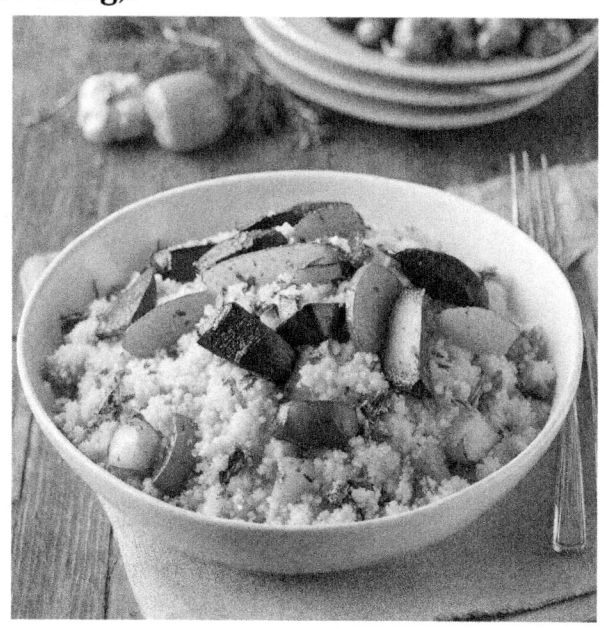

9. Caprese Sandwich

Ingredients:
- 4 ciabatta rolls, split
- 2 large tomatoes, sliced
- 8 ounces fresh mozzarella, sliced
- Fresh basil leaves
- Balsamic glaze
- Salt and pepper to taste

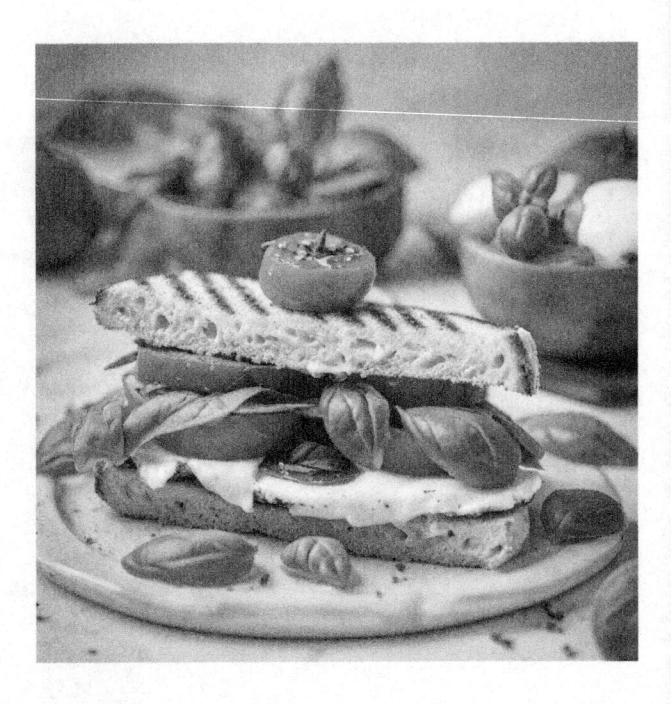

Instructions:
1. Layer each ciabatta roll with slices of tomato, mozzarella, and basil leaves.
2. Season with salt and pepper.
3. Drizzle with balsamic glaze.
4. Serve sandwiches immediately or press in a panini press for a grilled version.

Nutritional Information (per serving):
- Calories: 350
- Protein: 20 g
- Carbohydrates: 35 g
- Fat: 16 g
- Fiber: 2 g
- Sodium: 580 mg

Number of Servings: 4
Cooking Time: 10 minutes

10. Butternut Squash Risotto

Ingredients:
- 1 butternut squash, peeled and diced
- 1 tablespoon olive oil
- Salt and pepper to taste
- 1 onion, finely chopped
- 2 cups Arborio rice
- 6 cups chicken or vegetable broth, heated
- 1/2 cup grated Parmesan cheese
- 2 tablespoons unsalted butter

Instructions:
1. Preheat oven to 400°F (200°C). Toss butternut squash with olive oil, salt, and pepper. Roast for 25 minutes, until tender.
2. In a large pot, sauté onion in butter until translucent.
3. Add Arborio rice and stir to coat with butter. Begin adding broth, one cup at a time, stirring frequently, until each cup is absorbed before adding the next.
4. Once rice is creamy and al dente, stir in roasted butternut squash and Parmesan cheese.
5. Season with salt and pepper to taste, and serve warm.

Nutritional Information (per serving):
- Calories: 500
- Protein: 12 g
- Carbohydrates: 90 g
- Fat: 12 g
- Fiber: 5 g
- Sodium: 950 mg

Number of Servings: 4
Cooking Time: 50 minutes

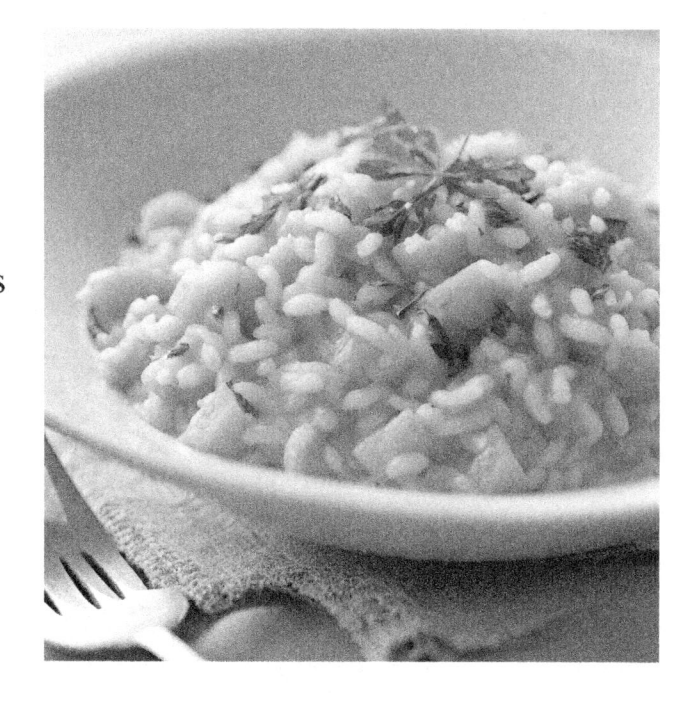

11. Mediterranean Chickpea Salad

Ingredients:
- 2 cups canned chickpeas, rinsed and drained
- 1 cucumber, diced
- 1 bell pepper, diced
- 1/2 red onion, thinly sliced
- 1/4 cup Kalamata olives, pitted and halved
- 1/4 cup feta cheese, crumbled
- 2 tablespoons olive oil
- 1 tablespoon red wine vinegar
- 1 teaspoon dried oregano
- Salt and pepper to taste

Instructions:
1. In a large bowl, combine chickpeas, cucumber, bell pepper, red onion, and olives.
2. In a small bowl, whisk together olive oil, red wine vinegar, oregano, salt, and pepper.
3. Pour the dressing over the salad and toss to combine.
4. Sprinkle feta cheese over the top before serving.

Nutritional Information (per serving):
- Calories: 250
- Protein: 8 g
- Carbohydrates: 25 g
- Fat: 13 g
- Fiber: 6 g
- Sodium: 300 mg

Number of Servings: 4
Cooking Time: 10 minutes (preparation time)

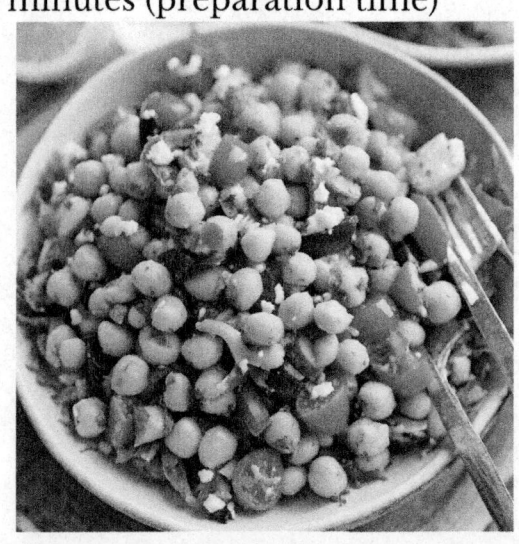

12. Grilled Chicken with Mango Salsa

Ingredients:
- 4 chicken breasts (4 oz each)
- 1 tablespoon olive oil
- Salt and pepper to taste
- 1 mango, peeled and diced
- 1/2 red bell pepper, diced
- 1/4 cup red onion, finely chopped
- 1 jalapeño, seeded and minced
- 1/4 cup fresh cilantro, chopped
- Juice of 1 lime

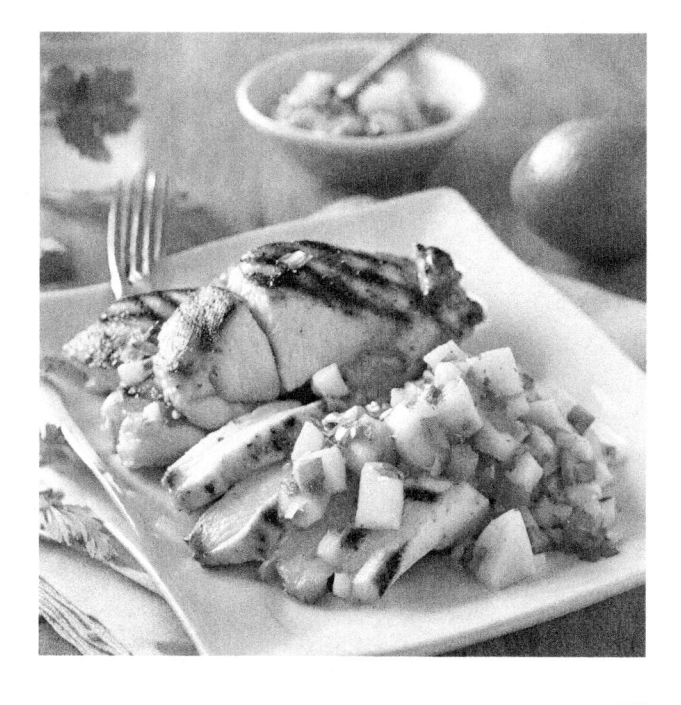

Instructions:
1. Preheat grill to medium-high heat.
2. Brush chicken breasts with olive oil and season with salt and pepper.
3. Grill chicken until cooked through, about 6-7 minutes per side.
4. While chicken is grilling, mix mango, bell pepper, onion, jalapeño, cilantro, and lime juice in a bowl to make the salsa.
5. Serve grilled chicken topped with mango salsa.

Nutritional Information (per serving):
- Calories: 250
- Protein: 26 g
- Carbohydrates: 15 g
- Fat: 9 g
- Fiber: 2 g
- Sodium: 200 mg

Number of Servings: 4
Cooking Time: 20 minutes

13. Baked Cod with Herb Crust

Ingredients:
- 4 cod fillets (4 oz each)
- 1/2 cup breadcrumbs
- 2 tablespoons grated Parmesan cheese
- 1 tablespoon fresh parsley, chopped
- 1 teaspoon dried thyme
- 1/4 teaspoon garlic powder
- 2 tablespoons olive oil
- Salt and pepper to taste

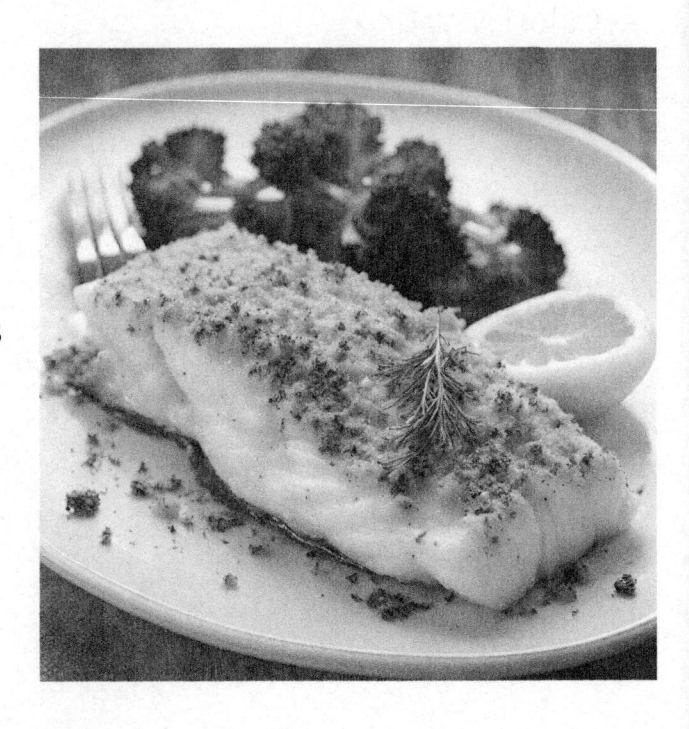

Instructions:
1. Preheat oven to 400°F (200°C).
2. In a small bowl, mix breadcrumbs, Parmesan, parsley, thyme, garlic powder, salt, and pepper.
3. Brush each cod fillet with olive oil and press the breadcrumb mixture onto the top of each fillet.
4. Place fillets on a baking sheet and bake for 12-15 minutes, until the crust is golden and the fish flakes easily with a fork.
5. Serve immediately.

Nutritional Information (per serving):
- Calories: 220
- Protein: 23 g
- Carbohydrates: 10 g
- Fat: 9 g
- Fiber: 1 g
- Sodium: 290 mg

Number of Servings: 4
Cooking Time: 20 minutes

14. Vegetable and Hummus Wraps
Ingredients:
- 4 whole wheat tortillas
- 1 cup hummus
- 1 cup mixed salad greens
- 1 carrot, julienned
- 1 cucumber, julienned
- 1 bell pepper, julienned
- 1/4 cup red onion, thinly sliced

Instructions:
1. Spread each tortilla with a layer of hummus.
2. Top with salad greens, carrot, cucumber, bell pepper, and red onion.
3. Roll up the tortillas tightly, slice in half, and serve.

Nutritional Information (per serving):
- Calories: 300
- Protein: 9 g
- Carbohydrates: 45 g
- Fat: 10 g
- Fiber: 8 g
- Sodium: 400 mg

Number of Servings: 4

Cooking Time: 10 minutes (preparation time)

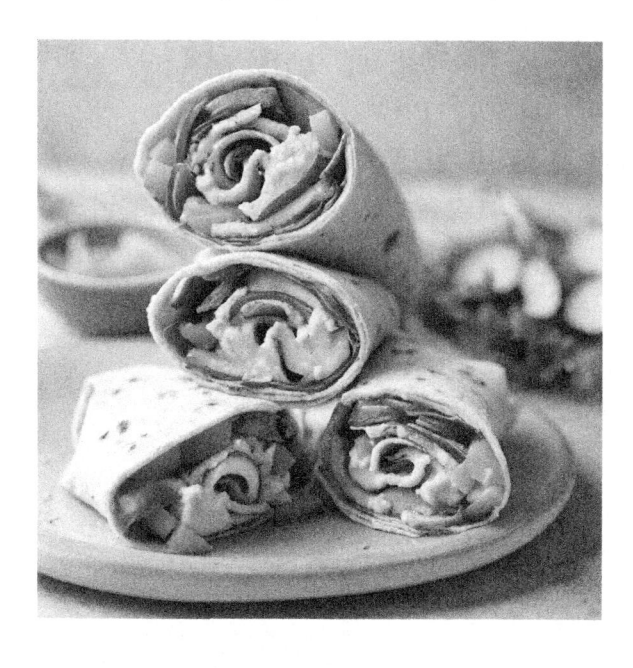

15. Rice Noodle Salad with Peanut Dressing

Ingredients:
- 8 oz rice noodles
- 1 cup shredded carrots
- 1 cup shredded red cabbage
- 1/2 cup thinly sliced bell peppers
- 1/4 cup chopped scallions
- 1/4 cup chopped cilantro
- **For the Peanut Dressing:**
    - 1/4 cup peanut butter
    - 2 tablespoons soy sauce (low sodium)
    - 1 tablespoon lime juice
    - 2 teaspoons honey
    - 1 teaspoon sesame oil
    - 1/4 teaspoon crushed red pepper flakes
    - Water to thin

Instructions:
1. Cook rice noodles according to package instructions, then rinse under cold water and drain.
2. In a large bowl, combine noodles, carrots, cabbage, bell peppers, scallions, and cilantro.
3. In a small bowl, whisk together peanut butter, soy sauce, lime juice, honey, sesame oil, and red pepper flakes. Add water as needed to reach desired consistency.
4. Pour dressing over noodle mixture and toss to coat.
5. Serve chilled or at room temperature.

Nutritional Information (per serving):
- Calories: 350
- Protein: 8 g
- Carbohydrates: 56 g
- Fat: 12 g
- Fiber: 3 g
- Sodium: 300 mg

Number of Servings: 4
Cooking Time: 20 minutes

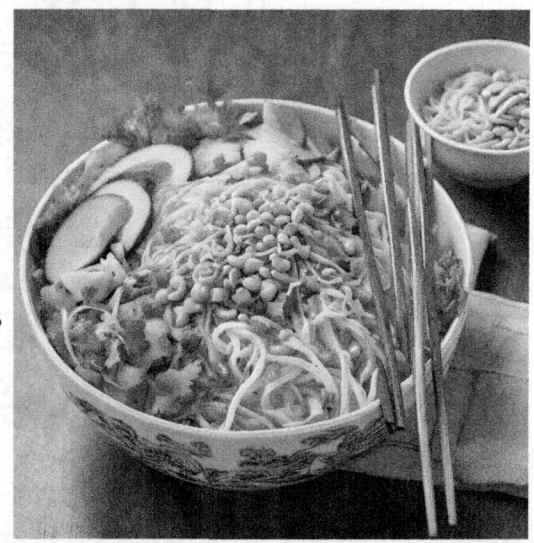

16. Roasted Turkey Breast Sandwich
Ingredients:
- 1 pound turkey breast, roasted and sliced
- 4 whole wheat sandwich buns
- 1/2 cup cranberry sauce
- 1/4 cup mayonnaise
- 1 cup arugula
- 1/2 red onion, thinly sliced

Instructions:
1. Spread cranberry sauce on the bottom half of each bun and mayonnaise on the top half.
2. Layer slices of turkey, arugula, and red onion on the bottom halves of the buns.
3. Top with the remaining bun halves and serve.

Nutritional Information (per serving):
- Calories: 400
- Protein: 25 g
- Carbohydrates: 45 g
- Fat: 15 g
- Fiber: 5 g
- Sodium: 550 mg

Number of Servings: 4

Cooking Time: 10 minutes (assembly after roasting)

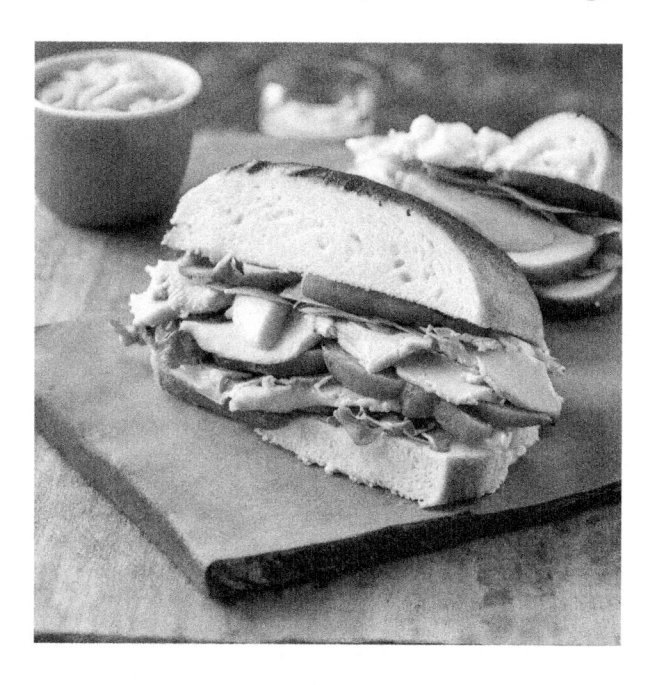

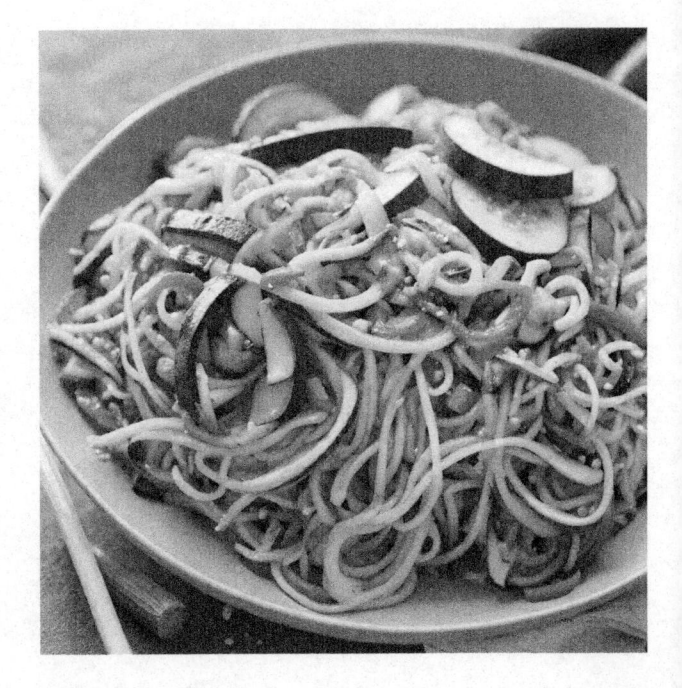

17. Zucchini Noodle Stir-Fry

Ingredients:
- 4 medium zucchini, spiralized into noodles
- 1 tablespoon olive oil
- 1 bell pepper, thinly sliced
- 1 carrot, julienned
- 1/2 red onion, thinly sliced
- 2 cloves garlic, minced
- 1 tablespoon soy sauce (low sodium)
- 1 tablespoon sesame seeds

Instructions:
1. Heat olive oil in a large skillet over medium heat.
2. Add bell pepper, carrot, and onion, and sauté until just tender.
3. Add garlic and cook for an additional minute.
4. Add zucchini noodles and soy sauce, cooking for 3-5 minutes until noodles are tender but still crisp.
5. Sprinkle with sesame seeds before serving.

Nutritional Information (per serving):
- Calories: 120
- Protein: 3 g
- Carbohydrates: 12 g
- Fat: 7 g
- Fiber: 3 g
- Sodium: 200 mg

Number of Servings: 4
Cooking Time: 20 minutes

18. Beef and Broccoli Stir-Fry

Ingredients:
- 1 lb beef sirloin, thinly sliced
- 4 cups broccoli florets
- 2 tablespoons vegetable oil
- 2 cloves garlic, minced
- 1/4 cup soy sauce (low sodium)
- 1 tablespoon cornstarch
- 1/2 cup beef broth (low sodium)
- 1 tablespoon sesame oil
- 1 teaspoon sugar

Instructions:
1. In a small bowl, mix the beef broth, soy sauce, cornstarch, sesame oil, and sugar until smooth.
2. Heat vegetable oil in a large skillet or wok over medium-high heat.
3. Add garlic and stir-fry briefly until fragrant.
4. Add beef and stir-fry until it is nearly cooked through.
5. Add broccoli and stir-fry for another 5 minutes until the vegetables are tender and the beef is fully cooked.
6. Pour the sauce mixture over the beef and broccoli, stirring well to coat. Cook for an additional 2-3 minutes until the sauce has thickened.
7. Serve hot with steamed rice if desired.

Nutritional Information (per serving):
- Calories: 300
- Protein: 25 g
- Carbohydrates: 15 g
- Fat: 15 g
- Fiber: 3 g
- Sodium: 550 mg

Number of Servings: 4
Cooking Time: 20 minutes

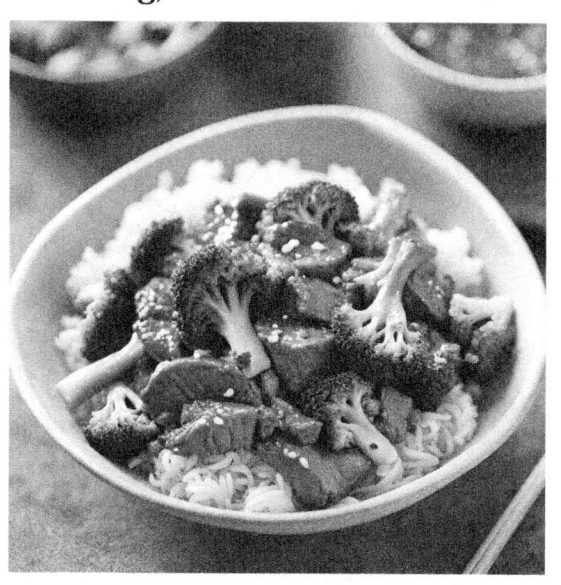

19. Greek Yogurt Chicken Salad

Ingredients:
- 2 cups cooked chicken breast, chopped
- 1/2 cup Greek yogurt
- 1/4 cup diced celery
- 1/4 cup diced apple
- 1/4 cup grapes, halved
- 2 tablespoons chopped walnuts
- 1 tablespoon lemon juice
- Salt and pepper to taste

Instructions:
1. In a large bowl, combine Greek yogurt, lemon juice, salt, and pepper.
2. Add chicken, celery, apple, grapes, and walnuts to the bowl and stir to combine.
3. Chill in the refrigerator for at least one hour before serving to allow flavors to meld.
4. Serve on lettuce leaves or as a sandwich filling.

Nutritional Information (per serving):
- Calories: 200
- Protein: 25 g
- Carbohydrates: 10 g
- Fat: 7 g
- Fiber: 2 g
- Sodium: 125 mg

Number of Servings: 4

Cooking Time: 10 minutes (plus chilling)

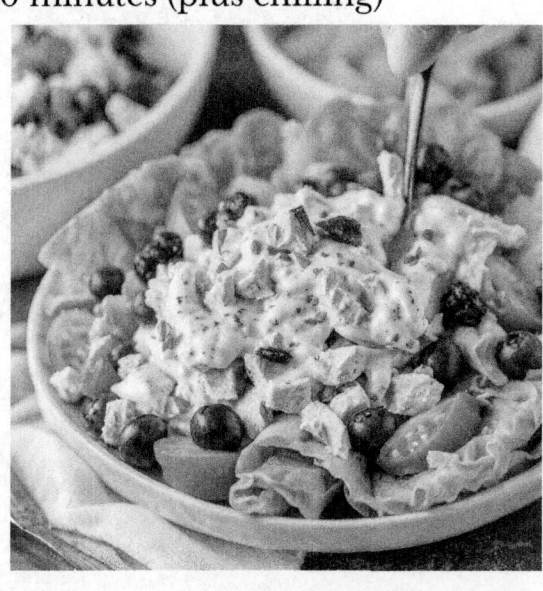

20. Balsamic Glazed Salmon

Ingredients:
- 4 salmon fillets (4 oz each)
- 1/4 cup balsamic vinegar
- 1 tablespoon honey
- 1 garlic clove, minced
- 1 tablespoon olive oil
- Salt and pepper to taste

Instructions:
1. Preheat your oven to 400°F (200°C).
2. In a small saucepan, combine balsamic vinegar, honey, and garlic. Simmer over medium heat until the mixture reduces by half and becomes syrupy, about 5-7 minutes.
3. Place salmon fillets on a baking sheet lined with parchment paper. Brush with olive oil and season with salt and pepper.
4. Bake the salmon for 12-15 minutes, then drizzle with the balsamic glaze and serve.

Nutritional Information (per serving):
- Calories: 280
- Protein: 23 g
- Carbohydrates: 7 g
- Fat: 17 g
- Fiber: 0 g
- Sodium: 75 mg

Number of Servings: 4
Cooking Time: 20 minutes

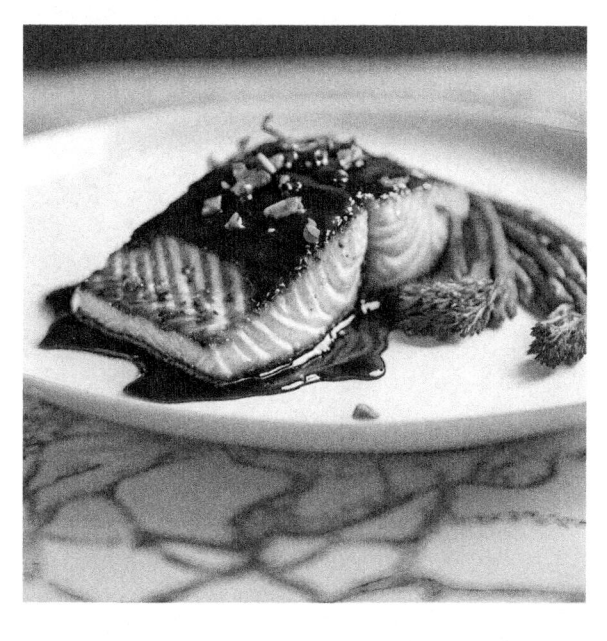

21. Portobello Mushroom Pizza

Ingredients:
- 4 large portobello mushroom caps, stems removed
- 1 cup marinara sauce
- 1 cup shredded mozzarella cheese
- 1/2 cup sliced bell peppers
- 1/2 cup sliced onions
- 1/4 cup sliced black olives
- 2 tablespoons olive oil
- Salt and pepper to taste

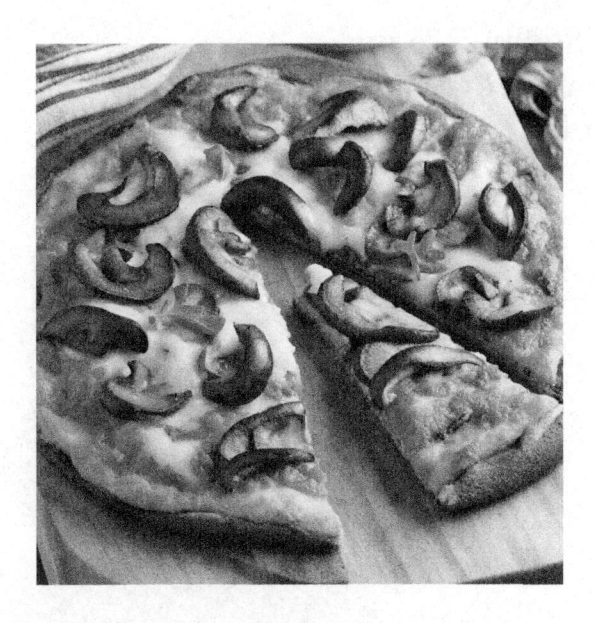

Instructions:
1. Preheat your oven to 375°F (190°C).
2. Brush both sides of the mushroom caps with olive oil and season with salt and pepper.
3. Place mushroom caps on a baking sheet, gill-side up.
4. Bake for 10 minutes to release some of their moisture.
5. Remove from the oven and top each mushroom with marinara sauce, mozzarella, bell peppers, onions, and olives.
6. Return to the oven and bake for another 10 minutes, or until the cheese is melted and bubbly.
7. Serve hot.

Nutritional Information (per serving):
- Calories: 220
- Protein: 10 g
- Carbohydrates: 10 g
- Fat: 16 g
- Fiber: 3 g
- Sodium: 460 mg

Number of Servings: 4
Cooking Time: 25 minutes

22. Sesame Chicken Salad

Ingredients:
- 1 lb chicken breast, cooked and shredded
- 4 cups mixed salad greens
- 1 carrot, shredded
- 1/2 cucumber, sliced
- 1/4 cup sliced almonds
- 2 tablespoons sesame seeds
- **For the dressing:**
    - 2 tablespoons soy sauce (low sodium)
    - 2 tablespoons rice vinegar
    - 1 tablespoon sesame oil
    - 1 tablespoon honey
    - 1 garlic clove, minced

Instructions:
1. In a large bowl, combine the cooked chicken, salad greens, carrot, cucumber, and sliced almonds.
2. In a small bowl, whisk together the soy sauce, rice vinegar, sesame oil, honey, and minced garlic to make the dressing.
3. Drizzle the dressing over the salad and toss to combine.
4. Sprinkle sesame seeds over the top before serving.

Nutritional Information (per serving):
- Calories: 290 Protein: 30 g Carbohydrates: 12 g Fat: 14 g
- Fiber: 3 g
- Sodium: 320 mg

Number of Servings: 4
Cooking Time: 15 minutes (if chicken is pre-cooked)

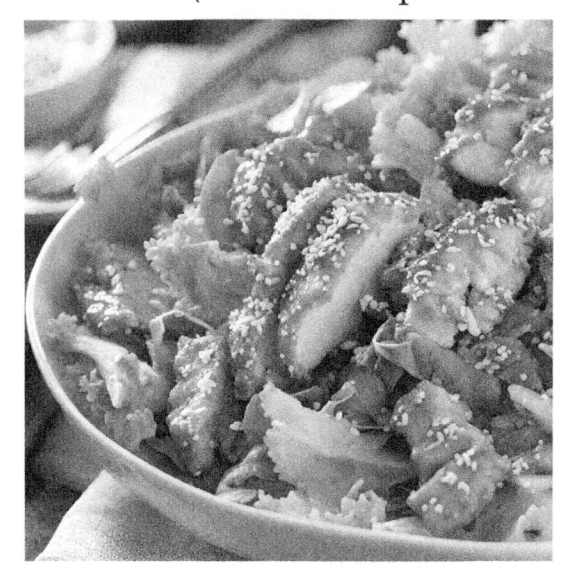

23. Cauliflower Rice Paella

Ingredients:
- 1 head cauliflower, grated into rice-sized pieces
- 1 tablespoon olive oil
- 1 onion, chopped
- 1 bell pepper, chopped
- 2 cloves garlic, minced
- 1/2 cup diced tomatoes
- 1/2 teaspoon saffron threads
- 1/2 teaspoon smoked paprika
- 1 cup low-sodium vegetable broth
- 1/2 lb shrimp, peeled and deveined
- 1/2 cup peas
- Salt and pepper to taste
- Lemon wedges for serving

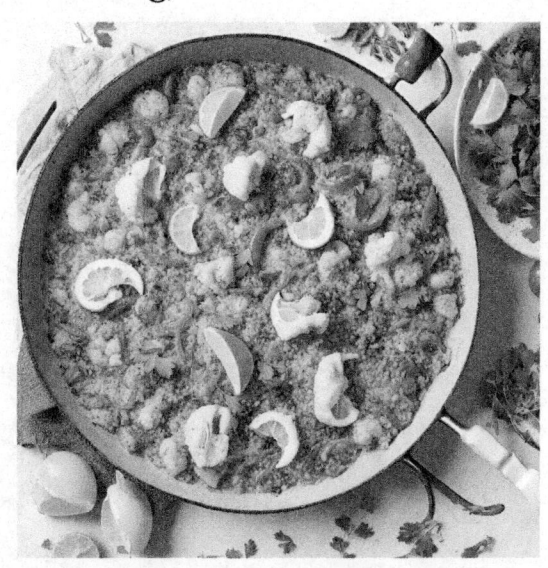

Instructions:
1. Heat olive oil in a large skillet over medium heat.
2. Add onion, bell pepper, and garlic and sauté until onions are translucent.
3. Stir in grated cauliflower, diced tomatoes, saffron, and smoked paprika.
4. Pour in vegetable broth and bring to a simmer.
5. Add shrimp and peas, cooking until shrimp are pink and cooked through.
6. Season with salt and pepper.
7. Serve hot with lemon wedges on the side.

Nutritional Information (per serving):
- Calories: 180
- Protein: 15 g
- Carbohydrates: 15 g
- Fat: 7 g
- Fiber: 4 g
- Sodium: 300 mg

Number of Servings: 4
Cooking Time: 30 minutes

24. Spaghetti Squash with Marinara Sauce

Ingredients:
- 1 large spaghetti squash
- 2 cups marinara sauce (low sodium)
- 1/2 cup grated Parmesan cheese
- 1 tablespoon olive oil
- Salt and pepper to taste
- Fresh basil for garnish

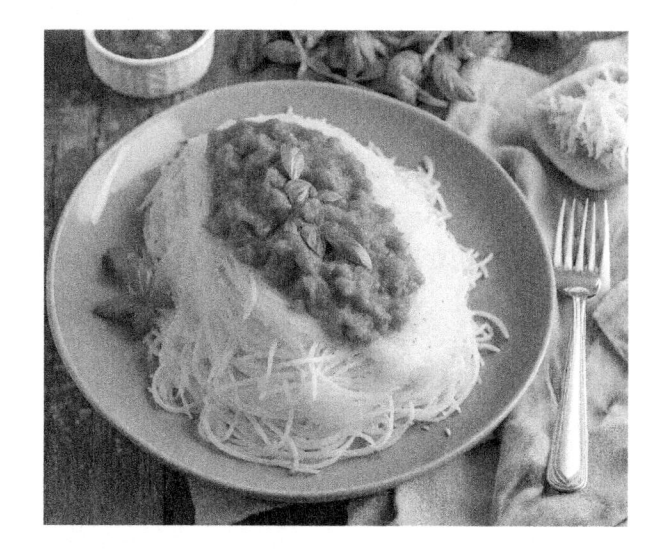

Instructions:
1. Preheat oven to 400°F (200°C).
2. Slice the spaghetti squash in half lengthwise and scoop out the seeds.
3. Brush the inside of each half with olive oil and season with salt and pepper.
4. Place squash halves cut side down on a baking sheet and roast for 40 minutes, until tender.
5. Use a fork to scrape the squash strands into a bowl.
6. Heat marinara sauce in a saucepan and pour over the squash.
7. Sprinkle with Parmesan cheese and garnish with fresh basil.
8. Serve hot.

Nutritional Information (per serving):
- Calories: 180
- Protein: 6 g
- Carbohydrates: 20 g
- Fat: 9 g
- Fiber: 4 g
- Sodium: 360 mg

Number of Servings: 4
Cooking Time: 50 minutes

25. Asian Cabbage Salad
Ingredients:
- 4 cups shredded cabbage
- 1 cup shredded carrots
- 1 red bell pepper, thinly sliced
- 1/4 cup chopped green onions
- 1/4 cup chopped cilantro
- **For the dressing:**
    - 3 tablespoons soy sauce (low sodium)
    - 2 tablespoons rice vinegar
    - 1 tablespoon sesame oil
    - 1 tablespoon honey
    - 1 teaspoon grated ginger

Instructions:
1. In a large salad bowl, combine cabbage, carrots, bell pepper, green onions, and cilantro.
2. In a small bowl, whisk together soy sauce, rice vinegar, sesame oil, honey, and ginger to create the dressing.
3. Pour the dressing over the salad and toss well to coat.
4. Chill in the refrigerator for at least 30 minutes before serving to allow flavors to meld.

Nutritional Information (per serving):
- Calories: 120
- Protein: 2 g
- Carbohydrates: 15 g
- Fat: 6 g
- Fiber: 3 g
- Sodium: 300 mg

Number of Servings: 4
Cooking Time: 10 minutes (plus chilling)

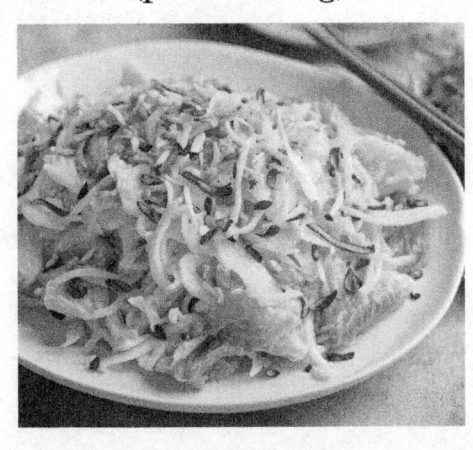

26. Tomato Basil Soup

Ingredients:
- 2 tablespoons olive oil
- 1 onion, chopped
- 2 cloves garlic, minced
- 1 can (28 ounces) crushed tomatoes
- 2 cups vegetable broth (low sodium)
- 1/4 cup fresh basil, chopped
- Salt and pepper to taste
- 1/2 cup heavy cream (optional)

Instructions:
1. Heat olive oil in a large pot over medium heat.
2. Add onion and garlic, sauté until onion is translucent.
3. Stir in crushed tomatoes and vegetable broth.
4. Bring to a boil, then reduce heat and simmer for 20 minutes.
5. Add chopped basil and season with salt and pepper.
6. Puree the soup with an immersion blender until smooth.
7. Stir in heavy cream if using, and heat through.
8. Serve hot.

Nutritional Information (per serving):
- Calories: 150 (without cream)
- Protein: 3 g
- Carbohydrates: 18 g
- Fat: 8 g (increases with cream)
- Fiber: 4 g
- Sodium: 250 mg

Number of Servings: 4
Cooking Time: 40 minutes

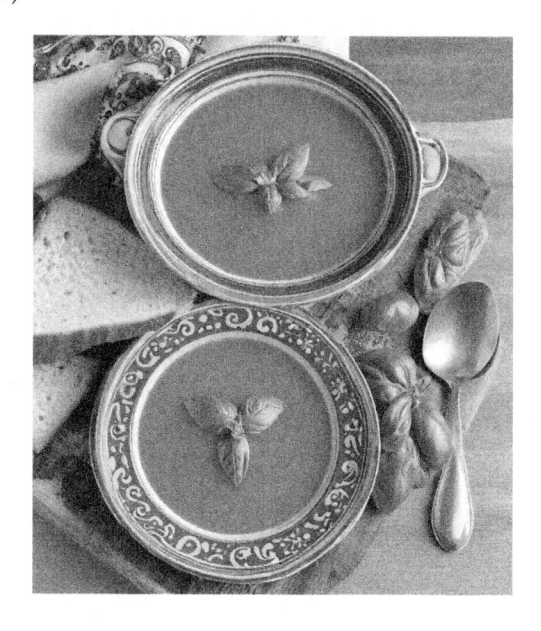

DINNER

1. Grilled Halibut with Lemon Herb Sauce
Ingredients:
- 4 halibut fillets (6 oz each)
- 2 tablespoons olive oil
- Salt and pepper to taste
- **For the Lemon Herb Sauce:**
    - 1/4 cup fresh parsley, chopped
    - 1/4 cup fresh basil, chopped
    - Juice of 2 lemons
    - 2 tablespoons olive oil
    - 1 garlic clove, minced
    - Salt to taste

Instructions:
1. Preheat the grill to medium-high heat.
2. Brush halibut fillets with olive oil and season with salt and pepper.
3. Grill the fillets for about 4-5 minutes on each side, until the fish flakes easily with a fork.
4. For the sauce, combine parsley, basil, lemon juice, olive oil, minced garlic, and a pinch of salt in a bowl. Mix well.
5. Serve the grilled halibut with the lemon herb sauce spooned over the top.

Nutritional Information (per serving):
- Calories: 280
- Protein: 35 g
- Carbohydrates: 3 g
- Fat: 14 g
- Fiber: 1 g
- Sodium: 120 mg

Number of Servings: 4
Cooking Time: 20 minutes

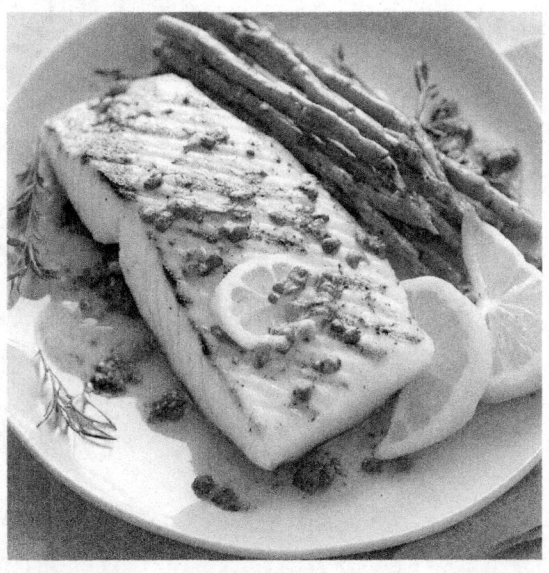

2. Roasted Chicken with Root Vegetables
Ingredients:
- 1 whole chicken (about 4 lbs)
- 3 carrots, peeled and cut into chunks
- 3 parsnips, peeled and cut into chunks
- 2 sweet potatoes, peeled and cut into chunks
- 3 tablespoons olive oil
- Salt and pepper to taste
- 1 teaspoon dried thyme

Instructions:
1. Preheat the oven to 400°F (200°C).
2. Place the chicken in a roasting pan.
3. Toss the carrots, parsnips, and sweet potatoes with olive oil, salt, pepper, and thyme. Arrange around the chicken.
4. Roast in the oven for about 1 hour and 20 minutes, or until the chicken's internal temperature reaches 165°F (75°C) and vegetables are tender.
5. Let the chicken rest for 10 minutes before carving. Serve with the roasted vegetables.

Nutritional Information (per serving):
- Calories: 560
- Protein: 44 g
- Carbohydrates: 32 g
- Fat: 28 g
- Fiber: 6 g
- Sodium: 340 mg

Number of Servings: 4
Cooking Time: 90 minutes

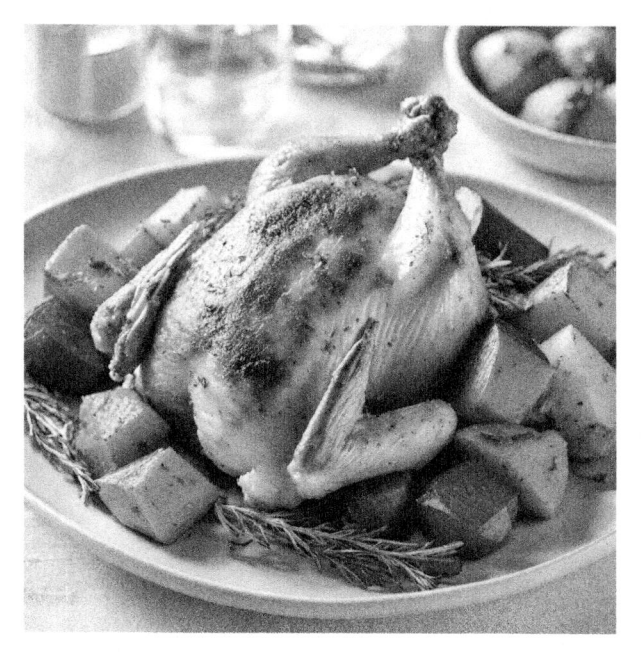

3. Pasta Primavera with Whole Wheat Spaghetti

Ingredients:
- 8 oz whole wheat spaghetti
- 1 zucchini, sliced
- 1 yellow squash, sliced
- 1 red bell pepper, julienned
- 1 cup cherry tomatoes, halved
- 2 cloves garlic, minced
- 2 tablespoons olive oil
- Salt and pepper to taste
- 1/4 cup grated Parmesan cheese
- 1/4 cup fresh basil, chopped

Instructions:
1. Cook spaghetti according to package instructions until al dente; drain.
2. Heat olive oil in a large skillet over medium heat. Add garlic, zucchini, squash, and bell pepper. Sauté for about 5 minutes.
3. Add cherry tomatoes and cook for an additional 3 minutes.
4. Toss the cooked vegetables with the spaghetti, Parmesan cheese, and fresh basil.
5. Season with salt and pepper and serve immediately.

Nutritional Information (per serving):
- Calories: 340
- Protein: 12 g
- Carbohydrates: 49 g
- Fat: 12 g
- Fiber: 8 g
- Sodium: 180 mg

Number of Servings: 4
Cooking Time: 30 minutes

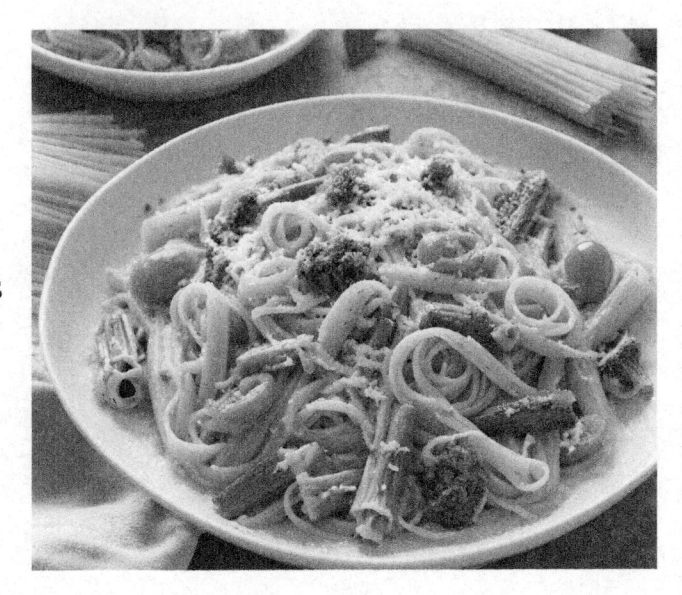

4. Baked Trout with Fennel and Citrus Salad

Ingredients:
- 4 trout fillets (6 oz each)
- 2 fennel bulbs, thinly sliced
- 1 orange, segmented
- 1 grapefruit, segmented
- 2 tablespoons olive oil
- Salt and pepper to taste
- 1 tablespoon fresh dill, chopped

Instructions:
1. Preheat the oven to 375°F (190°C).
2. Place trout fillets on a baking sheet lined with parchment paper. Drizzle with 1 tablespoon olive oil and season with salt and pepper.
3. Bake for 15-20 minutes, or until the trout is cooked through.
4. In a bowl, combine fennel, orange segments, grapefruit segments, remaining olive oil, and dill. Toss to mix.
5. Serve the baked trout topped with the fennel and citrus salad.

Nutritional Information (per serving):
- Calories: 290
- Protein: 32 g
- Carbohydrates: 15 g
- Fat: 12 g
- Fiber: 5 g
- Sodium: 150 mg

Number of Servings: 4
Cooking Time: 35 minutes

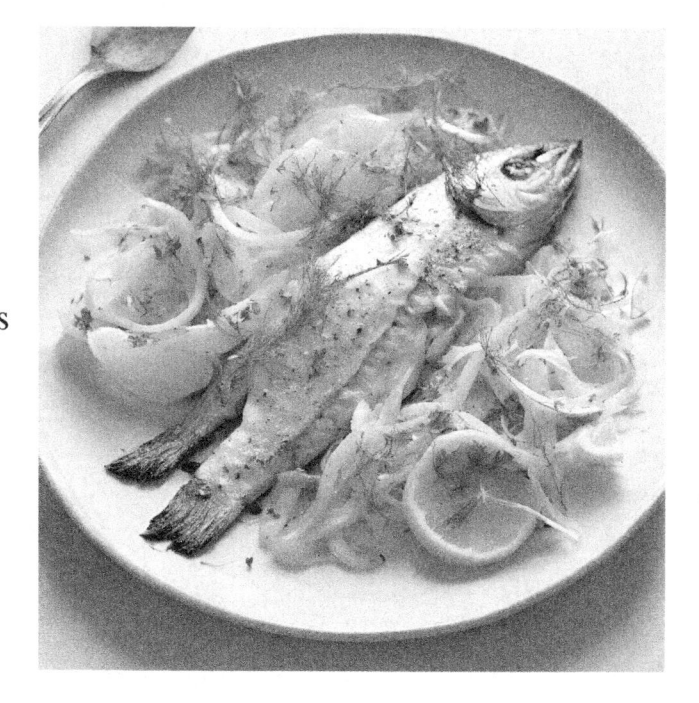

5. Vegetarian Chili

Ingredients:
- 1 tablespoon olive oil
- 1 onion, chopped
- 2 cloves garlic, minced
- 1 bell pepper, chopped
- 1 zucchini, chopped
- 2 carrots, peeled and chopped
- 1 can (15 oz) black beans, rinsed and drained
- 1 can (15 oz) kidney beans, rinsed and drained
- 2 cans (15 oz each) diced tomatoes
- 1 tablespoon chili powder
- 1 teaspoon cumin
- Salt and pepper to taste

Instructions:
1. Heat olive oil in a large pot over medium heat. Add onion and garlic and sauté until softened.
2. Add bell pepper, zucchini, and carrots. Cook for about 5 minutes, stirring occasionally.
3. Stir in black beans, kidney beans, diced tomatoes, chili powder, and cumin. Bring to a simmer.
4. Reduce heat and let simmer for 30 minutes, stirring occasionally.
5. Season with salt and pepper to taste.
6. Serve hot, garnished with sour cream or shredded cheese if desired.

Nutritional Information (per serving):
- Calories: 280
- Protein: 14 g
- Carbohydrates: 45 g
- Fat: 5 g
- Fiber: 12 g
- Sodium: 500 mg

Number of Servings: 6
Cooking Time: 45 minutes

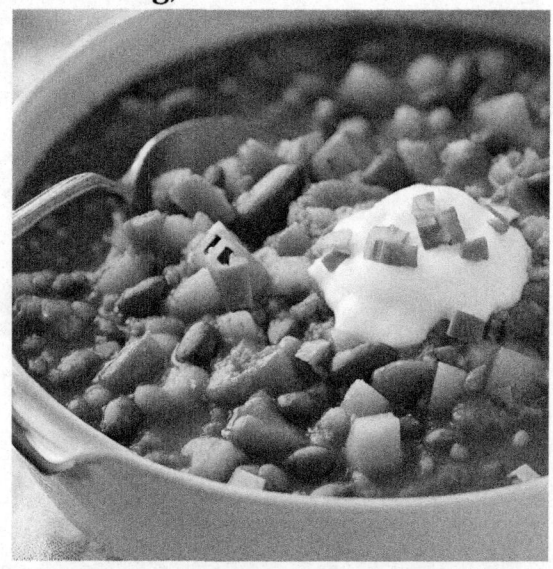

6. Stir-Fried Beef and Broccoli

Ingredients:
- 1 lb beef sirloin, thinly sliced
- 4 cups broccoli florets
- 2 tablespoons vegetable oil
- 2 cloves garlic, minced
- 1/4 cup soy sauce (low sodium)
- 1 tablespoon cornstarch
- 1/2 cup beef broth (low sodium)
- 1 tablespoon sesame oil
- 1 teaspoon sugar

Instructions:
1. In a small bowl, mix the beef broth, soy sauce, cornstarch, sesame oil, and sugar until smooth.
2. Heat vegetable oil in a large skillet or wok over medium-high heat.
3. Add garlic and stir-fry briefly until fragrant.
4. Add beef and stir-fry until it is nearly cooked through.
5. Add broccoli and stir-fry for another 5 minutes until the vegetables are tender and the beef is fully cooked.
6. Pour the sauce mixture over the beef and broccoli, stirring well to coat. Cook for an additional 2-3 minutes until the sauce has thickened.
7. Serve hot with steamed rice if desired.

Nutritional Information (per serving):
- Calories: 300
- Protein: 25 g
- Carbohydrates: 15 g
- Fat: 15 g
- Fiber: 3 g
- Sodium: 550 mg

Number of Servings: 4
Cooking Time: 20 minutes

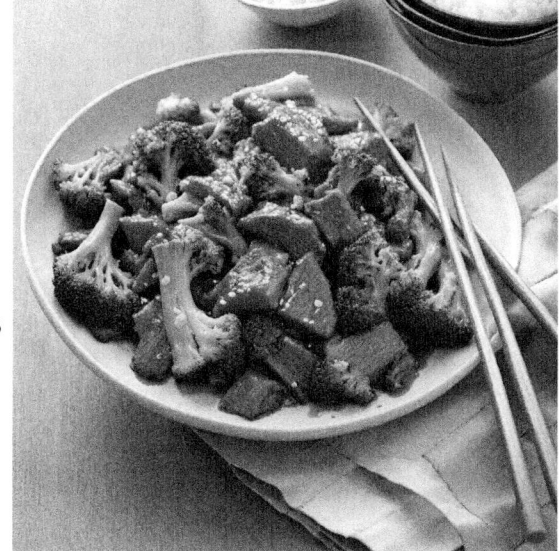

7. Lemon Garlic Shrimp with Asparagus

Ingredients:
- 1 lb large shrimp, peeled and deveined
- 1 lb asparagus, trimmed
- 2 tablespoons olive oil
- 3 cloves garlic, minced
- Juice of 1 lemon
- Zest of 1 lemon
- Salt and pepper to taste

Instructions:
1. Preheat your oven to 400°F (200°C).
2. Place shrimp and asparagus on a large baking sheet. Drizzle with olive oil and sprinkle with minced garlic, lemon zest, and lemon juice. Season with salt and pepper.
3. Toss everything together to coat and spread out in an even layer.
4. Bake for 8-10 minutes, or until the shrimp are pink and opaque.
5. Serve immediately.

Nutritional Information (per serving):
- Calories: 230
- Protein: 24 g
- Carbohydrates: 7 g
- Fat: 12 g
- Fiber: 3 g
- Sodium: 200 mg

Number of Servings: 4
Cooking Time: 20 minutes

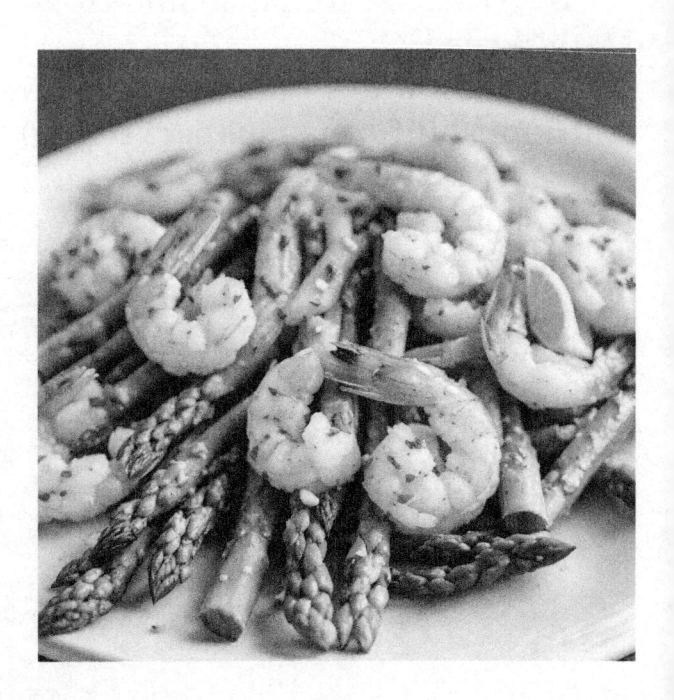

8. Cauliflower Steak with Tahini Sauce

Ingredients:
- 2 large heads cauliflower
- 3 tablespoons olive oil
- Salt and pepper to taste
- **For the Tahini Sauce:**
  - 1/4 cup tahini
  - 1 garlic clove, minced
  - Juice of 1 lemon
  - 2 tablespoons water
  - Salt to taste

Instructions:
1. Preheat the oven to 425°F (220°C).
2. Slice each cauliflower head into thick "steaks" approximately 1 inch thick.
3. Place cauliflower steaks on a baking sheet, brush with olive oil, and season with salt and pepper.
4. Roast in the oven for about 20-25 minutes, flipping halfway through, until tender and golden.
5. For the sauce, whisk together tahini, garlic, lemon juice, water, and salt until smooth.
6. Drizzle tahini sauce over roasted cauliflower steaks and serve.

Nutritional Information (per serving):
- Calories: 210
- Protein: 5 g
- Carbohydrates: 15 g
- Fat: 16 g
- Fiber: 5 g
- Sodium: 75 mg

Number of Servings: 4
Cooking Time: 35 minutes

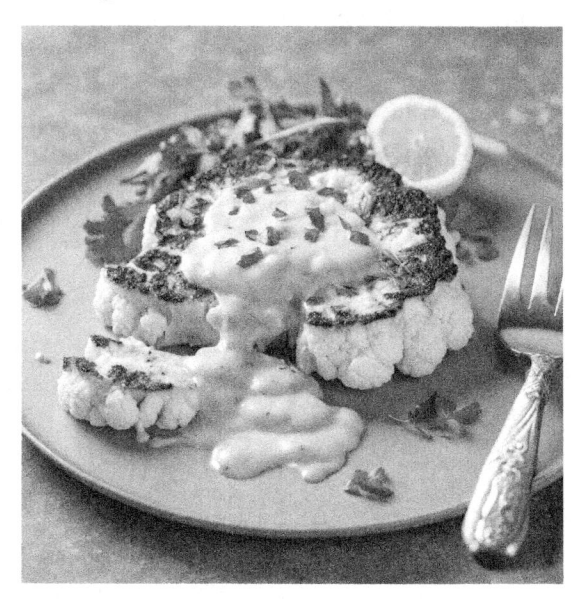

9. Grilled Pork Chops with Apple Slaw

Ingredients:
- 4 pork chops (1-inch thick)
- Salt and pepper to taste
- 2 tablespoons olive oil
- **For the Apple Slaw:**
    - 2 apples, julienned
    - 1/4 head cabbage, shredded
    - Juice of 1 lemon
    - 1 tablespoon honey
    - 2 tablespoons olive oil
    - Salt and pepper to taste

Instructions:
1. Preheat grill to medium-high heat.
2. Season pork chops with salt, pepper, and brush with olive oil.
3. Grill for about 5-6 minutes per side or until the internal temperature reaches 145°F (63°C).
4. For the slaw, mix together apples, cabbage, lemon juice, honey, and olive oil in a bowl. Season with salt and pepper.
5. Serve grilled pork chops topped with apple slaw.

Nutritional Information (per serving):
- Calories: 370
- Protein: 29 g
- Carbohydrates: 22 g
- Fat: 18 g
- Fiber: 4 g
- Sodium: 180 mg

Number of Servings: 4
Cooking Time: 25 minutes

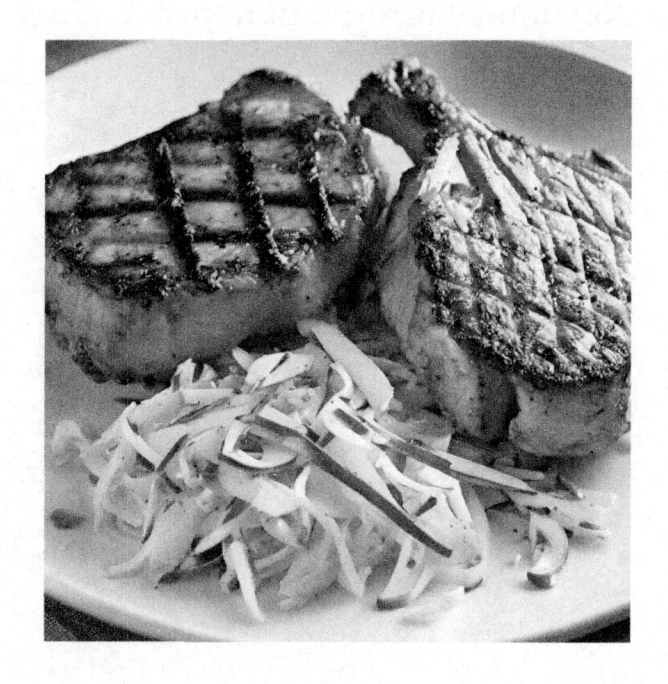

10. Seared Scallops with Cauliflower Puree

Ingredients:
- 12 large scallops
- 1 head cauliflower, cut into florets
- 2 tablespoons olive oil
- 1/2 cup milk
- Salt and pepper to taste

Instructions:
1. Steam the cauliflower until very tender, about 10 minutes.
2. In a blender, puree the steamed cauliflower with milk, salt, and pepper until smooth.
3. Heat olive oil in a pan over high heat. Season scallops with salt and pepper.
4. Sear scallops for about 1-2 minutes per side until golden and just cooked through.
5. Serve scallops over a bed of cauliflower puree.

Nutritional Information (per serving):
- Calories: 210
- Protein: 18 g
- Carbohydrates: 10 g
- Fat: 12 g
- Fiber: 3 g
- Sodium: 340 mg

Number of Servings: 4
Cooking Time: 30 minutes

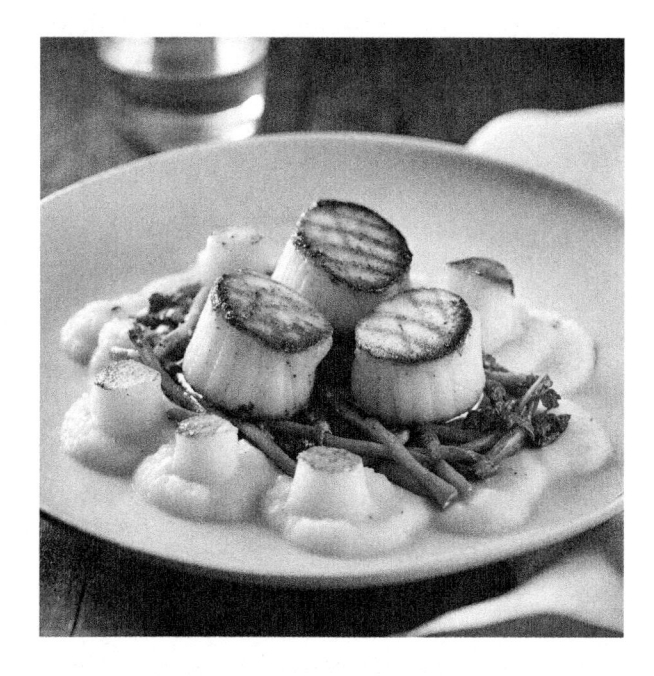

11. Baked Tilapia with Lemon Parsley Quinoa

Ingredients:
- 4 tilapia fillets (6 oz each)
- 2 tablespoons olive oil
- Juice and zest of 1 lemon
- Salt and pepper to taste
- 1 cup quinoa
- 2 cups water
- 1/4 cup chopped parsley

Instructions:
1. Preheat your oven to 400°F (200°C).
2. Place tilapia fillets on a baking sheet lined with parchment paper. Drizzle with olive oil and lemon juice, then season with lemon zest, salt, and pepper.
3. Bake in the preheated oven for 12-15 minutes, until fish flakes easily with a fork.
4. Meanwhile, rinse quinoa under cold water. Bring water to a boil in a saucepan, add quinoa, and reduce to a simmer. Cover and cook until all water is absorbed, about 15 minutes.
5. Stir chopped parsley into the cooked quinoa and season with salt and pepper.
6. Serve baked tilapia over the lemon parsley quinoa.

Nutritional Information (per serving):
- Calories: 290
- Protein: 28 g
- Carbohydrates: 23 g
- Fat: 10 g
- Fiber: 3 g
- Sodium: 75 mg

Number of Servings: 4
Cooking Time: 30 minutes

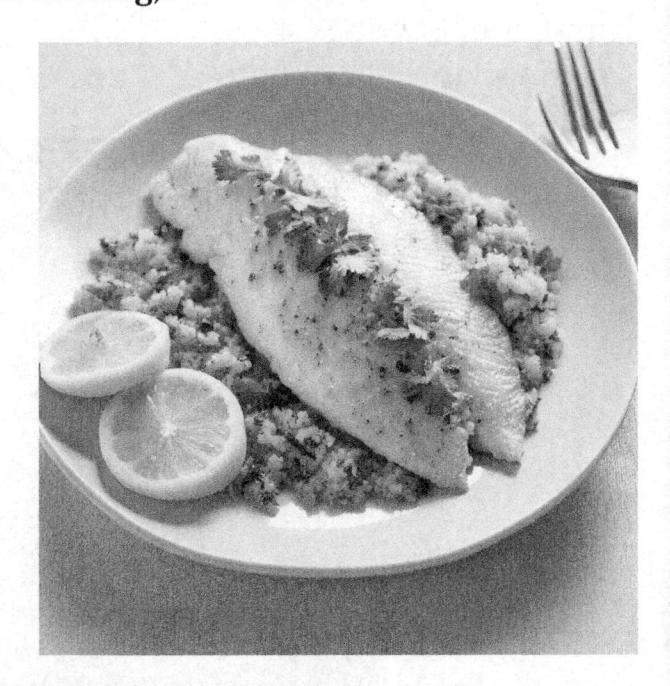

12. Chicken Piccata

Ingredients:
- 4 boneless, skinless chicken breasts (6 oz each)
- 1/4 cup all-purpose flour
- Salt and pepper to taste
- 2 tablespoons olive oil
- 1/4 cup lemon juice
- 1/2 cup chicken broth (low sodium)
- 1/4 cup capers
- 2 tablespoons chopped parsley
- 2 tablespoons unsalted butter

Instructions:
1. Flatten chicken breasts to an even thickness with a meat mallet.
2. Season flour with salt and pepper and dredge chicken breasts in the flour, shaking off the excess.
3. Heat olive oil in a large skillet over medium-high heat. Cook chicken until golden and cooked through, about 4 minutes per side. Remove from the skillet and set aside.
4. Add lemon juice, chicken broth, and capers to the skillet. Bring to a simmer.
5. Return chicken to the skillet and simmer for 5 minutes. Stir in butter and parsley until butter is melted.
6. Serve chicken with the sauce drizzled over the top.

Nutritional Information (per serving):
- Calories: 320
- Protein: 26 g
- Carbohydrates: 8 g
- Fat: 20 g
- Fiber: 0.5 g
- Sodium: 320 mg

Number of Servings: 4
Cooking Time: 30 minutes

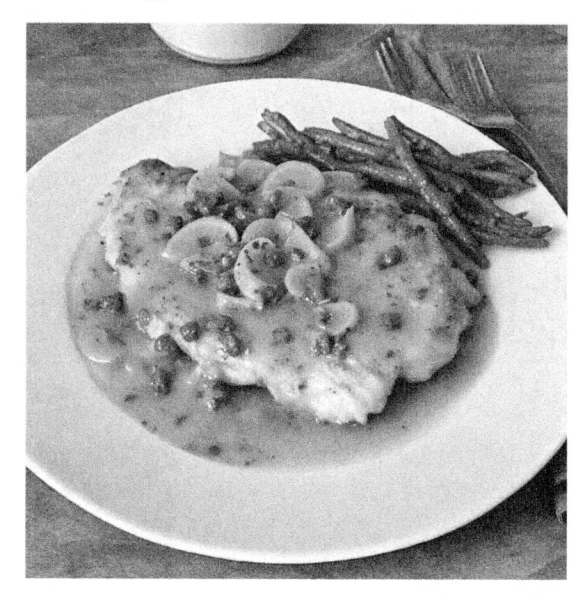

13. Vegetable Paella
Ingredients:
- 2 tablespoons olive oil
- 1 onion, chopped
- 1 red bell pepper, chopped
- 2 cloves garlic, minced
- 1 cup Arborio rice
- 3 cups vegetable broth (low sodium)
- 1 teaspoon saffron threads
- 1/2 teaspoon smoked paprika
- 1 cup frozen peas
- 1/2 cup chopped tomatoes
- Salt and pepper to taste
- 1/4 cup chopped parsley

Instructions:
1. Heat olive oil in a large skillet over medium heat. Add onion, bell pepper, and garlic, and sauté until soft.
2. Stir in rice, saffron, and paprika. Cook for 2 minutes.
3. Add vegetable broth and bring to a boil. Reduce heat to low and simmer, covered, for 20 minutes.
4. Stir in peas and tomatoes and cook for an additional 5 minutes, until rice is tender and liquid is absorbed.
5. Season with salt and pepper, garnish with parsley, and serve.

Nutritional Information (per serving):
- Calories: 290
- Protein: 6 g
- Carbohydrates: 52 g
- Fat: 7 g
- Fiber: 4 g
- Sodium: 300 mg

Number of Servings: 4
Cooking Time: 35 minutes

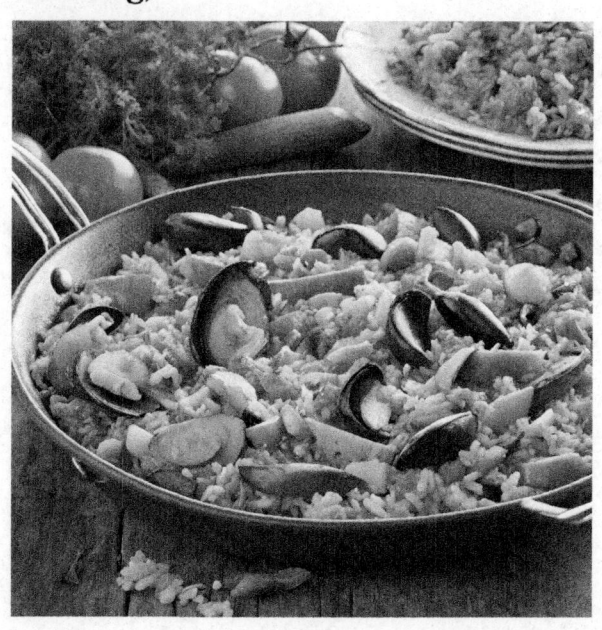

14. Moroccan Spiced Carrot Soup

Ingredients:
- 2 tablespoons olive oil
- 1 onion, chopped
- 1 pound carrots, peeled and chopped
- 4 cups vegetable broth (low sodium)
- 2 teaspoons ground cumin
- 1 teaspoon ground cinnamon
- 1/2 teaspoon ground ginger
- Salt and pepper to taste
- 1/2 cup coconut milk

Instructions:
1. Heat olive oil in a large pot over medium heat. Add onion and sauté until translucent.
2. Add carrots and cook for 5 minutes.
3. Stir in cumin, cinnamon, and ginger, then add vegetable broth.
4. Bring to a boil, then reduce heat and simmer for 30 minutes, until carrots are very tender.
5. Puree the soup in a blender or with an immersion blender until smooth.
6. Stir in coconut milk and season with salt and pepper.
7. Serve hot, garnished with a swirl of coconut milk or fresh herbs if desired.

Nutritional Information (per serving):
- Calories: 180
- Protein: 3 g
- Carbohydrates: 20 g
- Fat: 11 g
- Fiber: 4 g
- Sodium: 300 mg

Number of Servings: 4
Cooking Time: 45 minutes

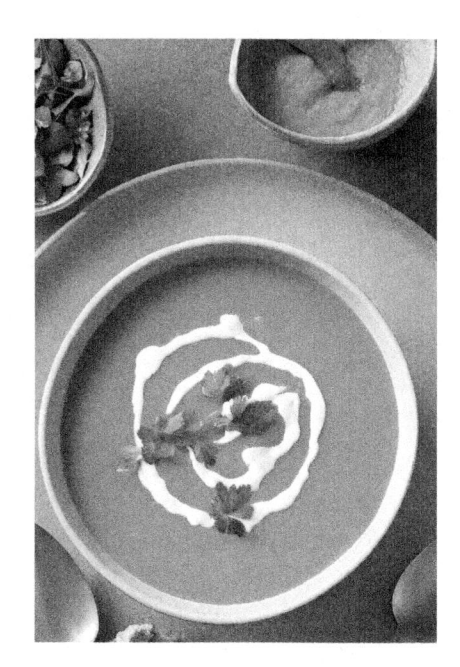

15. Cod with Parsley Pesto and Steamed Vegetables

Ingredients:
- 4 cod fillets (6 oz each)
- 1 cup fresh parsley
- 1/4 cup almonds
- 2 cloves garlic
- 1/4 cup olive oil
- Juice of 1 lemon
- Salt and pepper to taste
- 2 cups mixed vegetables (broccoli, carrots, snap peas)

Instructions:
1. For the parsley pesto, blend parsley, almonds, garlic, olive oil, and lemon juice in a food processor until smooth. Season with salt and pepper.
2. Season cod fillets with salt and pepper. Place in a baking dish.
3. Spread a layer of parsley pesto over each fillet.
4. Bake in a preheated 400°F (200°C) oven for 12-15 minutes, until fish flakes easily.
5. Steam vegetables until tender, about 7-10 minutes.
6. Serve cod with steamed vegetables on the side.

Nutritional Information (per serving):
- Calories: 280
- Protein: 28 g
- Carbohydrates: 8 g
- Fat: 16 g
- Fiber: 3 g
- Sodium: 200 mg

Number of Servings: 4
Cooking Time: 30 minutes

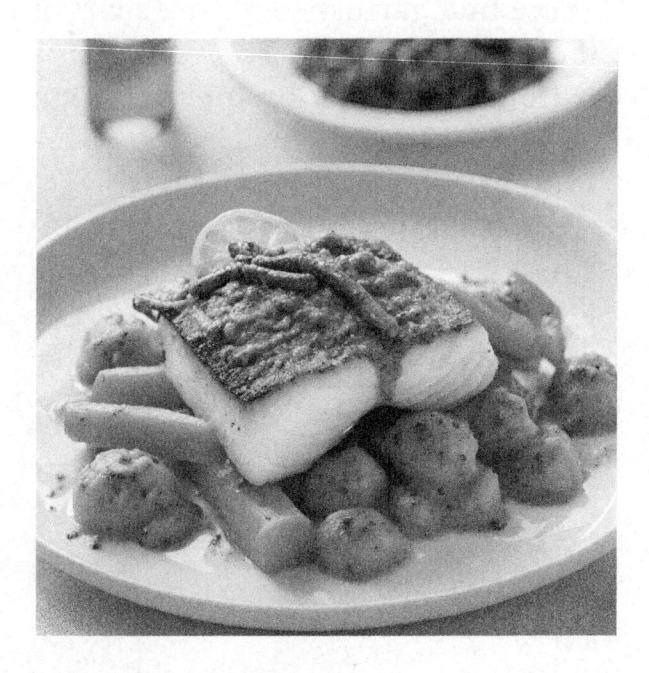

16. Turkey Stuffed Bell Peppers

Ingredients:
- 4 large bell peppers, tops cut off and seeds removed
- 1 lb ground turkey
- 1 cup cooked quinoa
- 1 onion, chopped
- 1 cup diced tomatoes
- 1 clove garlic, minced
- 1 teaspoon cumin
- 1/2 teaspoon paprika
- Salt and pepper to taste
- 1/2 cup shredded low-fat cheese

Instructions:
1. Preheat oven to 375°F (190°C).
2. In a skillet over medium heat, cook ground turkey and onion until the meat is browned and onions are soft.
3. Stir in garlic, cumin, paprika, and diced tomatoes. Cook for 5 minutes.
4. Mix in cooked quinoa and season with salt and pepper.
5. Fill bell peppers with the turkey mixture and place them upright in a baking dish.
6. Top each pepper with shredded cheese.
7. Bake for 25-30 minutes, until peppers are tender and cheese is melted.
8. Serve hot.

Nutritional Information (per serving):
- Calories: 310
- Protein: 26 g
- Carbohydrates: 24 g
- Fat: 12 g
- Fiber: 5 g
- Sodium: 320 mg

Number of Servings: 4
Cooking Time: 55 minutes

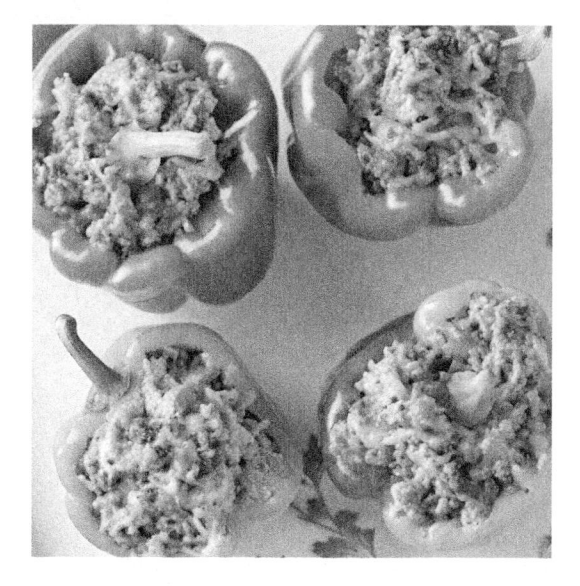

17. Squash and Chickpea Moroccan Stew

Ingredients:
- 1 tablespoon olive oil
- 1 onion, chopped
- 2 cloves garlic, minced
- 1 butternut squash, peeled and cubed
- 1 can (15 oz) chickpeas, rinsed and drained
- 1 can (15 oz) diced tomatoes
- 2 cups vegetable broth
- 1 teaspoon ground cumin
- 1 teaspoon ground coriander
- 1/2 teaspoon ground cinnamon
- Salt to taste
- Chopped cilantro for garnish

Instructions:
1. Heat olive oil in a large pot over medium heat. Add onion and garlic, and sauté until onion is translucent.
2. Add butternut squash, chickpeas, tomatoes, and vegetable broth.
3. Stir in cumin, coriander, and cinnamon.
4. Bring to a boil, then reduce heat and simmer for 20-25 minutes, until squash is tender.
5. Season with salt. Serve hot, garnished with chopped cilantro.

Nutritional Information (per serving):
- Calories: 220
- Protein: 7 g
- Carbohydrates: 37 g
- Fat: 5 g
- Fiber: 9 g
- Sodium: 300 mg

Number of Servings: 4
Cooking Time: 45 minutes

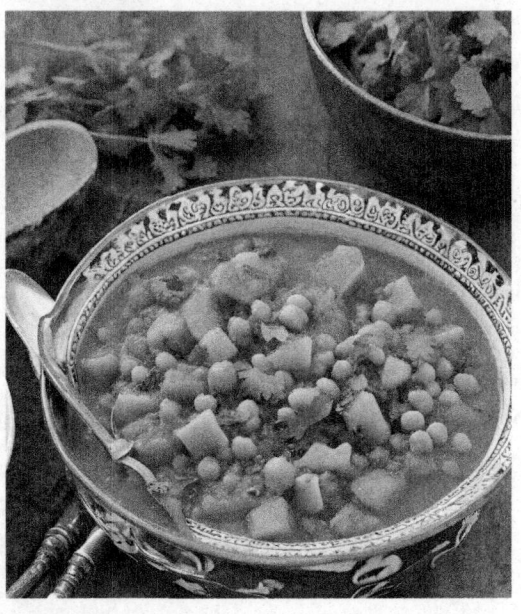

18. Herbed Lamb Chops with Spinach Salad

Ingredients:
- 8 lamb chops
- 2 tablespoons olive oil
- 1 tablespoon rosemary, minced
- 1 tablespoon thyme, minced
- Salt and pepper to taste
- **For the Spinach Salad:**
    - 4 cups fresh spinach
    - 1/4 cup sliced almonds
    - 1/4 cup dried cranberries
    - 2 tablespoons balsamic vinegar
    - 1 tablespoon olive oil

Instructions:
1. Rub lamb chops with olive oil, rosemary, thyme, salt, and pepper.
2. Grill lamb chops over medium-high heat for about 3-4 minutes per side, until desired doneness.
3. For the salad, toss spinach, almonds, and cranberries with balsamic vinegar and olive oil.
4. Serve lamb chops with spinach salad on the side.

Nutritional Information (per serving):
- Calories: 350
- Protein: 24 g
- Carbohydrates: 10 g
- Fat: 24 g
- Fiber: 3 g
- Sodium: 200 mg

Number of Servings: 4
Cooking Time: 20 minutes

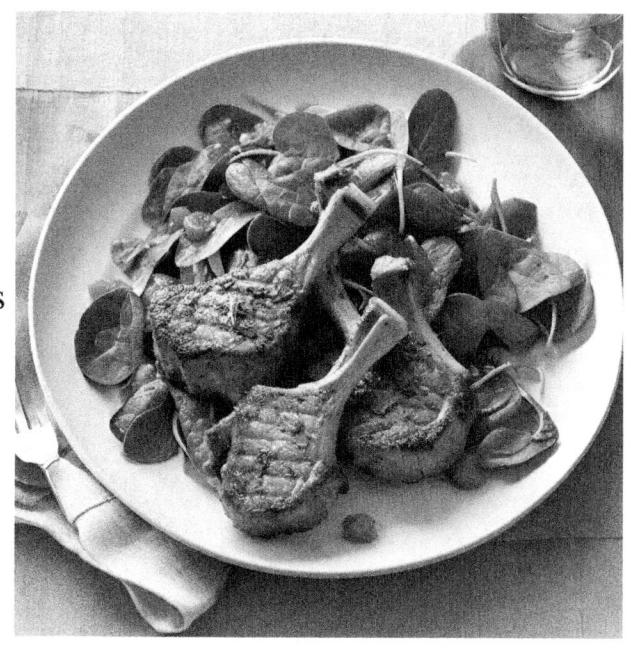

19. Tofu and Vegetable Curry

Ingredients:
- 1 block firm tofu, cubed
- 2 tablespoons vegetable oil
- 1 onion, chopped
- 2 cloves garlic, minced
- 1 tablespoon ginger, minced
- 1 bell pepper, chopped
- 1 zucchini, chopped
- 1 tablespoon curry powder
- 1 can (14 oz) coconut milk
- Salt to taste

Instructions:
1. Heat oil in a large skillet over medium heat. Add onion, garlic, and ginger, and sauté until onion is soft.
2. Add bell pepper and zucchini, cooking for another 5 minutes.
3. Stir in curry powder and cook for 1 minute.
4. Add tofu and coconut milk. Bring to a simmer and cook for 10 minutes.
5. Season with salt. Serve hot over cooked rice or with naan bread.

Nutritional Information (per serving):
- Calories: 320
- Protein: 12 g
- Carbohydrates: 15 g
- Fat: 24 g
- Fiber: 3 g
- Sodium: 80 mg

Number of Servings: 4
Cooking Time: 30 minutes

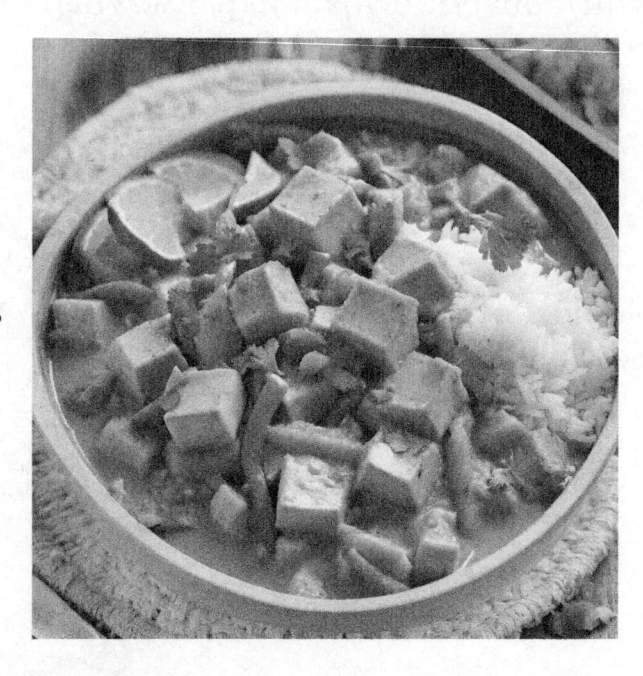

20. Basil Pesto Pasta with Chicken

Ingredients:
- 8 oz whole wheat spaghetti
- 2 boneless, skinless chicken breasts
- 1 cup basil leaves
- 1/4 cup pine nuts
- 2 cloves garlic
- 1/4 cup grated Parmesan cheese
- 1/4 cup olive oil
- Salt and pepper to taste

Instructions:
1. Cook pasta according to package directions; drain.
2. Grill chicken breasts until fully cooked, then slice.
3. In a food processor, combine basil, pine nuts, garlic, and Parmesan. Pulse until coarsely chopped.
4. Stream in olive oil while processing until smooth. Season pesto with salt and pepper.
5. Toss cooked pasta with pesto and top with sliced chicken.
6. Serve immediately.

Nutritional Information (per serving):
- Calories: 550
- Protein: 32 g
- Carbohydrates: 45 g
- Fat: 27 g
- Fiber: 6 g
- Sodium: 220 mg

Number of Servings: 4
Cooking Time: 30 minutes

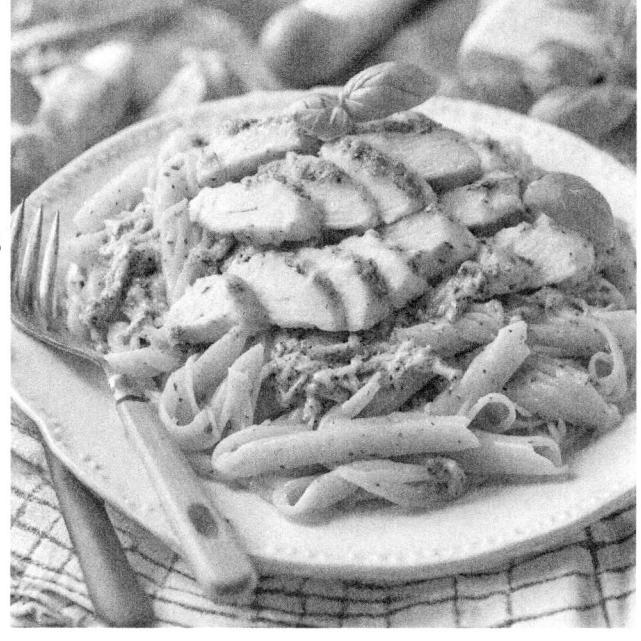

21. Roasted Duck with Orange Sauce

Ingredients:
- 1 whole duck (about 4-5 lbs)
- Salt and pepper to taste
- **For the Orange Sauce:**
    - Juice and zest of 2 oranges
    - 1 tablespoon sugar
    - 1/2 cup chicken broth
    - 2 tablespoons vinegar
    - 1 teaspoon cornstarch dissolved in 1 tablespoon water

Instructions:
1. Preheat oven to 350°F (175°C).
2. Season the duck with salt and pepper, and place it breast side up on a rack in a roasting pan.
3. Roast for about 2 hours, or until the internal temperature reaches 165°F (74°C) and the skin is golden and crispy.
4. For the orange sauce, combine orange juice, zest, sugar, chicken broth, and vinegar in a saucepan. Bring to a simmer.
5. Add the cornstarch mixture, and stir until the sauce thickens slightly.
6. Carve the duck and serve with the orange sauce drizzled over the top.

Nutritional Information (per serving):
- Calories: 560
- Protein: 43 g
- Carbohydrates: 11 g
- Fat: 38 g
- Fiber: 0 g
- Sodium: 300 mg

Number of Servings: 4
Cooking Time: 2 hours 15 minutes

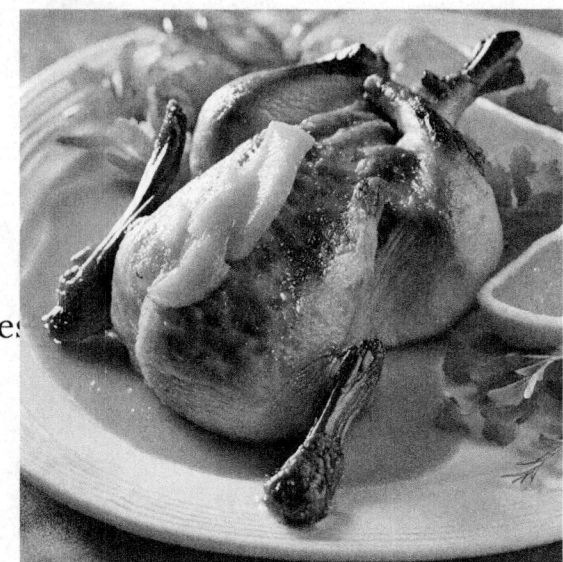

22. Minted Pea and Barley Risotto

Ingredients:
- 1 cup pearled barley
- 1 tablespoon olive oil
- 1 onion, finely chopped
- 4 cups vegetable broth
- 1 cup fresh or frozen peas
- 1/4 cup fresh mint, chopped
- 1/4 cup Parmesan cheese, grated
- Salt and pepper to taste

Instructions:
1. Heat olive oil in a large saucepan over medium heat. Add onion and sauté until translucent.
2. Add barley and stir to coat with oil.
3. Begin adding broth, 1 cup at a time, stirring frequently until each addition is absorbed before adding the next.
4. When barley is tender and creamy, stir in peas and cook until heated through.
5. Remove from heat, stir in mint and Parmesan. Season with salt and pepper.
6. Serve hot.

Nutritional Information (per serving):
- Calories: 350
- Protein: 12 g
- Carbohydrates: 55 g
- Fat: 9 g
- Fiber: 10 g
- Sodium: 450 mg

Number of Servings: 4
Cooking Time: 55 minutes

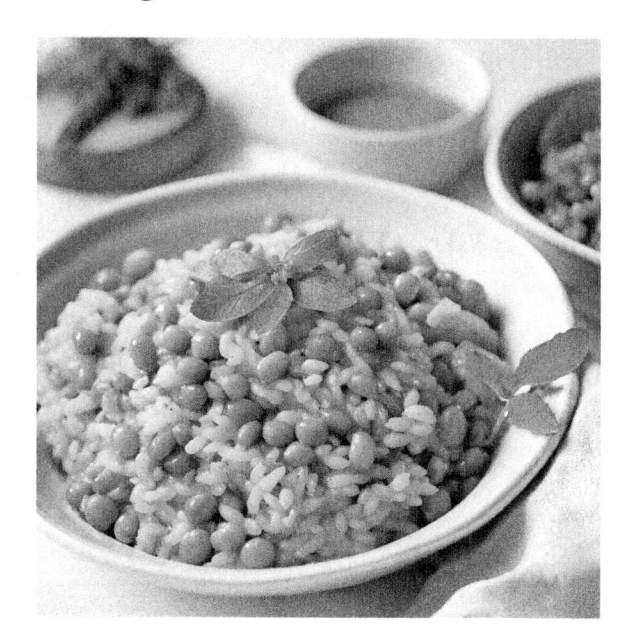

23. Asian Glazed Salmon

Ingredients:
- 4 salmon fillets (6 oz each)
- 1/4 cup soy sauce (low sodium)
- 2 tablespoons honey
- 1 tablespoon ginger, grated
- 1 garlic clove, minced
- 1 tablespoon sesame oil
- 1 tablespoon sesame seeds
- 1 green onion, thinly sliced

Instructions:
1. Preheat oven to 400°F (200°C).
2. In a small bowl, whisk together soy sauce, honey, ginger, garlic, and sesame oil.
3. Place salmon fillets in a baking dish and pour the marinade over them.
4. Bake for 15-20 minutes, or until salmon is cooked through and flakes easily with a fork.
5. Sprinkle with sesame seeds and green onion before serving.

Nutritional Information (per serving):
- Calories: 340
- Protein: 23 g
- Carbohydrates: 9 g
- Fat: 23 g
- Fiber: 0 g
- Sodium: 530 mg

Number of Servings: 4
Cooking Time: 30 minutes

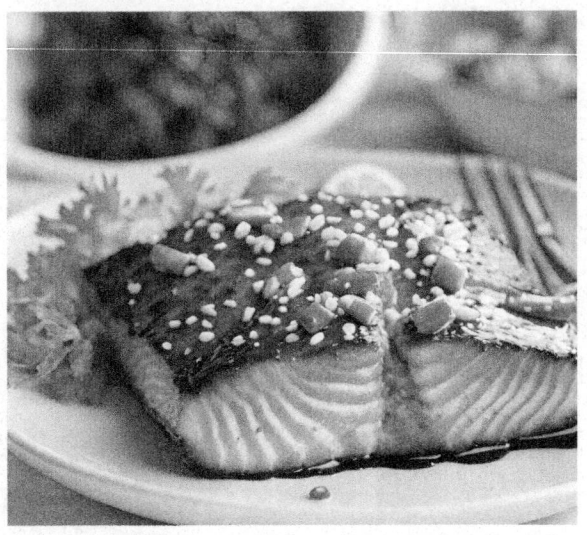

24. Chickpea and Spinach Stew
Ingredients:
- 2 tablespoons olive oil
- 1 onion, chopped
- 2 cloves garlic, minced
- 1 teaspoon ground cumin
- 1/2 teaspoon smoked paprika
- 1 can (15 oz) chickpeas, drained and rinsed
- 1 can (14 oz) diced tomatoes
- 4 cups fresh spinach
- Salt and pepper to taste

Instructions:
1. Heat olive oil in a large pot over medium heat.
2. Add onion and garlic and sauté until onion is translucent.
3. Stir in cumin and paprika, cook for another minute.
4. Add chickpeas and tomatoes, bring to a simmer.
5. Stir in spinach until wilted. Season with salt and pepper.
6. Serve hot, possibly with crusty bread.

Nutritional Information (per serving):
- Calories: 220
- Protein: 8 g
- Carbohydrates: 30
- Fat: 7 g
- Fiber: 8 g
- Sodium: 430 mg

Number of Servings: 4
Cooking Time: 30 minutes

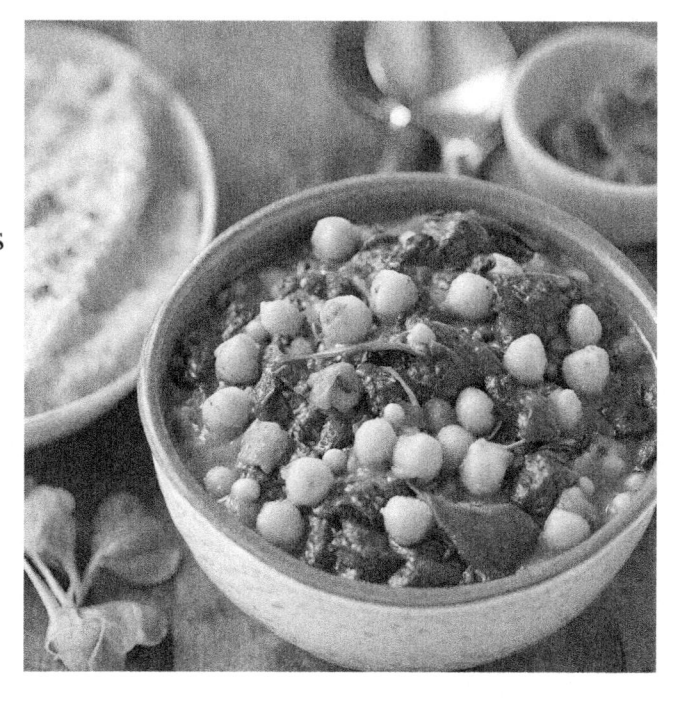

25. Cauliflower and Turmeric Soup

Ingredients:
- 1 tablespoon olive oil
- 1 onion, chopped
- 2 cloves garlic, minced
- 1 head cauliflower, chopped into florets
- 1 teaspoon turmeric
- 4 cups vegetable broth (low sodium)
- Salt and pepper to taste
- 1/2 cup coconut milk

Instructions:
1. Heat olive oil in a large pot over medium heat. Add onion and garlic, sauté until soft.
2. Add cauliflower and turmeric, stirring to coat the florets evenly.
3. Pour in vegetable broth, bring to a boil, then reduce heat and simmer for 20 minutes, or until cauliflower is tender.
4. Use an immersion blender to puree the soup until smooth.
5. Stir in coconut milk, season with salt and pepper, and heat through.
6. Serve hot, garnished with a swirl of coconut milk or fresh herbs if desired.

Nutritional Information (per serving):
- Calories: 160
- Protein: 4 g
- Carbohydrates: 15 g
- Fat: 10 g
- Fiber: 4 g
- Sodium: 300 mg

Number of Servings: 4
Cooking Time: 35 minutes

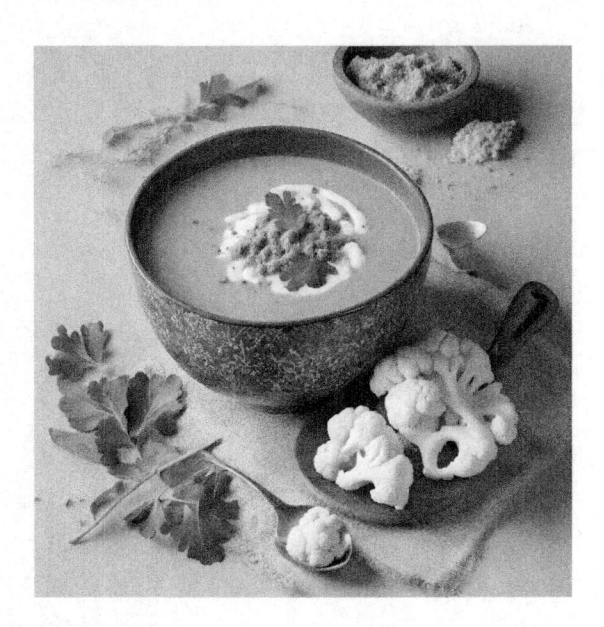

26. Grilled Shrimp and Polenta

Ingredients:
- 1 lb large shrimp, peeled and deveined
- 2 tablespoons olive oil
- 1 teaspoon paprika
- Salt and pepper to taste
- 1 cup polenta (cornmeal)
- 4 cups water
- 1 tablespoon butter
- 1/4 cup grated Parmesan cheese

Instructions:
1. Preheat grill to medium-high heat.
2. Toss shrimp with olive oil, paprika, salt, and pepper.
3. Grill shrimp for 2-3 minutes on each side, until pink and cooked through.
4. Meanwhile, bring water to a boil in a saucepan. Gradually whisk in polenta. Reduce heat and simmer, stirring frequently, until polenta is thick and creamy, about 15-20 minutes.
5. Stir in butter and Parmesan cheese until melted and incorporated. Season with salt and pepper.
6. Serve grilled shrimp over creamy polenta.

Nutritional Information (per serving):
- Calories: 380
- Protein: 25 g
- Carbohydrates: 30 g
- Fat: 18 g
- Fiber: 2 g
- Sodium: 600 mg

Number of Servings: 4
Cooking Time: 30 minutes

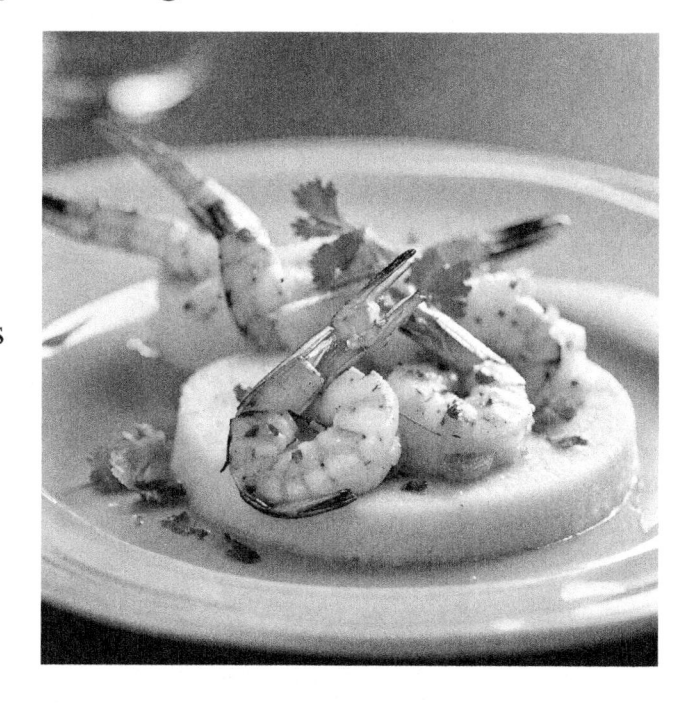

27. Lemon Rosemary Grilled Swordfish

Ingredients:
- 4 swordfish steaks (6 oz each)
- 2 tablespoons olive oil
- Juice of 1 lemon
- 1 tablespoon chopped fresh rosemary
- Salt and pepper to taste

Instructions:
1. Preheat grill to high heat.
2. In a small bowl, combine olive oil, lemon juice, rosemary, salt, and pepper.
3. Brush swordfish steaks with the lemon-rosemary mixture.
4. Grill swordfish for 4-5 minutes per side, or until the fish is opaque and flakes easily with a fork.
5. Serve immediately, with extra lemon wedges if desired.

Nutritional Information (per serving):
- Calories: 280
- Protein: 23 g
- Carbohydrates: 1 g
- Fat: 20 g
- Fiber: 0 g
- Sodium: 125 mg

Number of Servings: 4
Cooking Time: 20 minutes

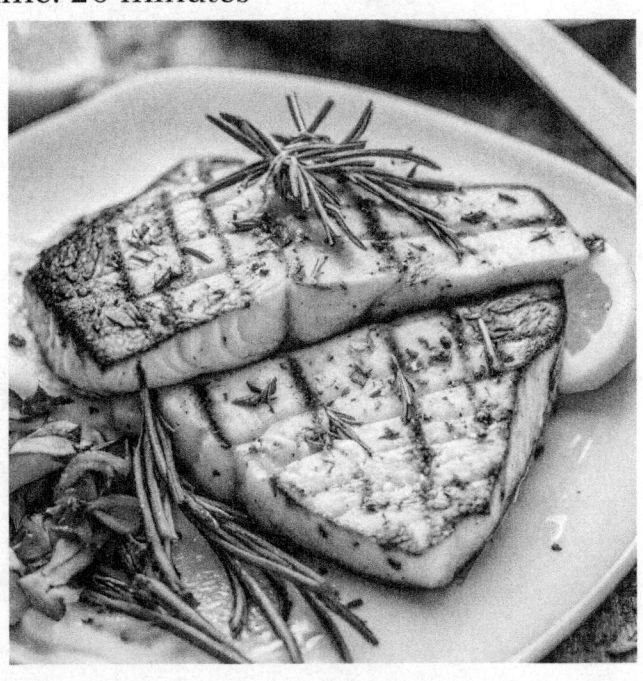

DESSERTS

1. Zucchini Brownies
Ingredients:
- 1/2 cup vegetable oil
- 1 cup sugar
- 2 teaspoons vanilla extract
- 1 cup flour
- 1/4 cup unsweetened cocoa powder
- 1 and 1/2 teaspoons baking soda
- 1 teaspoon salt
- 2 cups shredded zucchini
- 1/2 cup chopped walnuts (optional)

Instructions:
1. Preheat oven to 350°F (175°C). Grease a 9x9 inch baking pan.
2. In a large bowl, mix together oil, sugar, and vanilla until well blended.
3. Combine flour, cocoa, baking soda, and salt; stir into the sugar mixture.
4. Fold in zucchini and walnuts. Spread evenly into the prepared pan.
5. Bake for 25-30 minutes in the preheated oven, until brownies spring back when gently touched.
6. Let cool in pan before cutting into squares.

Nutritional Information (per serving):
- Calories: 210
- Protein: 2 g
- Carbohydrates: 28 g
- Fat: 10 g
- Fiber: 2 g
- Sodium: 220 mg

Number of Servings: 16
Cooking Time: 30 minutes

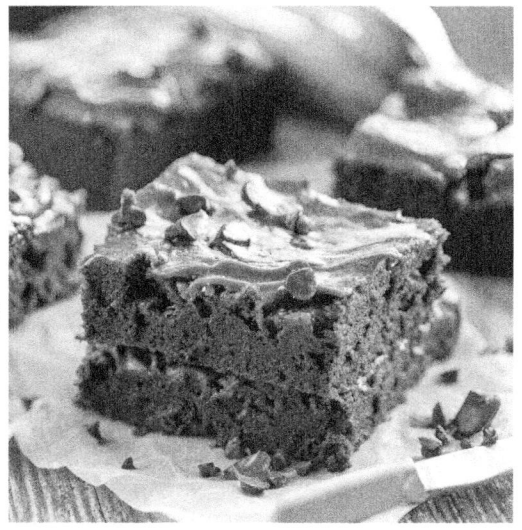

2. Caramelized Pear Bread Pudding

Ingredients:
- 3 ripe pears, peeled and sliced
- 1/4 cup brown sugar
- 1 teaspoon cinnamon
- 2 tablespoons butter
- 4 cups cubed day-old bread
- 2 cups milk
- 3 eggs
- 1 teaspoon vanilla extract
- 1/2 cup granulated sugar

Instructions:
1. Preheat oven to 350°F (175°C). Grease a 9x13 inch baking dish.
2. In a skillet over medium heat, melt butter. Add pears, brown sugar, and cinnamon. Cook until pears are caramelized, about 10 minutes.
3. In a large bowl, whisk together milk, eggs, vanilla, and granulated sugar.
4. Stir in bread cubes and let soak for a few minutes.
5. Stir in caramelized pears and pour into prepared baking dish.
6. Bake for 45 minutes, or until set and golden brown.
7. Serve warm.

Nutritional Information (per serving):
- Calories: 180
- Protein: 4 g
- Carbohydrates: 32 g
- Fat: 5 g
- Fiber: 2 g
- Sodium: 150 mg

Number of Servings: 8
Cooking Time: 55 minutes

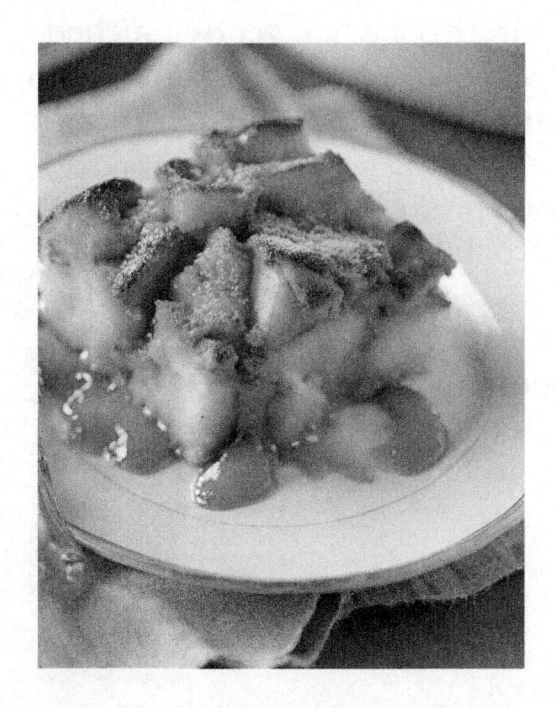

3. Key Lime Pie with Almond Crust

Ingredients:
- **For the crust:**
    - 1 and 1/2 cups almond flour
    - 1/4 cup melted butter
    - 1 tablespoon sugar
- **For the filling:**
    - 1 can (14 oz) sweetened condensed milk
    - 1/2 cup key lime juice
    - 1 teaspoon lime zest
    - 2 eggs

Instructions:
1. Preheat oven to 350°F (175°C).
2. Mix almond flour, melted butter, and sugar in a bowl. Press into the bottom and up the sides of a 9-inch pie dish.
3. Bake crust for 10 minutes; remove from oven.
4. Whisk together sweetened condensed milk, key lime juice, lime zest, and eggs until smooth.
5. Pour into prebaked crust and return to oven.
6. Bake for 15 minutes, until filling is set.
7. Chill in the refrigerator for at least 2 hours before serving.

Nutritional Information (per serving):
- Calories: 320
- Protein: 7 g
- Carbohydrates: 28 g
- Fat: 20 g
- Fiber: 2 g
- Sodium: 180 mg

Number of Servings: 8
Cooking Time: 25 minutes plus chilling

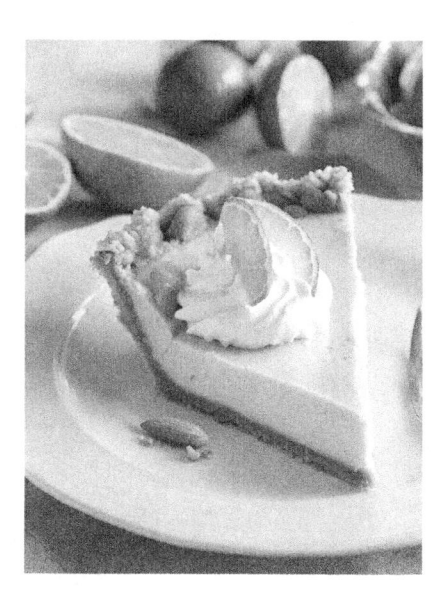

4. Balsamic Strawberries with Whipped Cream

Ingredients:
- 1 pound fresh strawberries, hulled and sliced
- 2 tablespoons balsamic vinegar
- 1 tablespoon sugar
- 1 cup heavy cream
- 2 tablespoons powdered sugar

Instructions:
1. In a bowl, combine strawberries, balsamic vinegar, and sugar. Let marinate for 30 minutes.
2. In a separate bowl, whip the heavy cream and powdered sugar until stiff peaks form.
3. Serve marinated strawberries topped with whipped cream.

Nutritional Information (per serving):
- Calories: 200
- Protein: 1 g
- Carbohydrates: 15 g
- Fat: 15 g
- Fiber: 2 g
- Sodium: 20 mg

Number of Servings: 4

Cooking Time: 10 minutes (plus marinating)

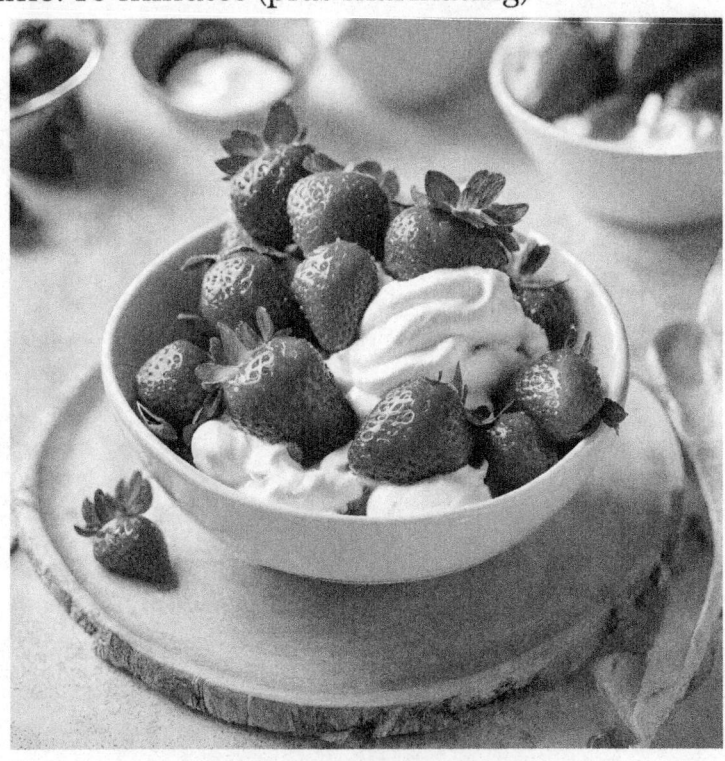

5. Vanilla Bean Panna Cotta

Ingredients:
- 2 cups heavy cream
- 1/2 cup sugar
- 1 vanilla bean, split lengthwise
- 1 packet gelatin (about 2 teaspoons)
- 3 tablespoons cold water

Instructions:
1. Place cold water in a small bowl and sprinkle gelatin over it. Let stand to soften gelatin.
2. In a saucepan, combine heavy cream and sugar. Scrape seeds from the vanilla bean into the cream and add the bean pod.
3. Heat over medium heat until hot but not boiling. Remove from heat and discard the vanilla bean pod.
4. Add the softened gelatin to the hot cream mixture and stir until completely dissolved.
5. Pour into serving dishes or molds. Refrigerate until set, about 4 hours.
6. Serve chilled.

Nutritional Information (per serving):
- Calories: 310
- Protein: 3 g
- Carbohydrates: 25 g
- Fat: 22 g
- Fiber: 0 g
- Sodium: 55 mg

Number of Servings: 4

Cooking Time: 15 minutes (plus 4 hours to set)

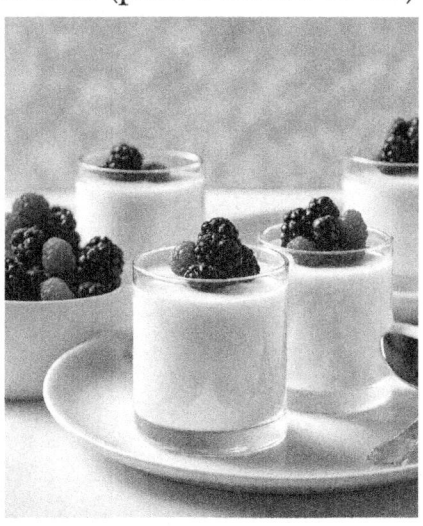

6. Cherry Sorbet

Ingredients:
- 4 cups fresh cherries, pitted
- 1/2 cup sugar
- 1 cup water
- Juice of 1 lemon

Instructions:
1. In a saucepan, combine water and sugar. Heat over medium heat, stirring until sugar dissolves. Let cool.
2. In a blender, puree cherries with the cooled syrup and lemon juice until smooth.
3. Strain through a fine mesh sieve to remove solids.
4. Chill the mixture thoroughly, then freeze in your ice cream maker according to the manufacturer's instructions.
5. Transfer to a container and freeze until firm.

Nutritional Information (per serving):
- Calories: 180
- Protein: 1 g
- Carbohydrates: 45 g
- Fat: 0 g
- Fiber: 2 g
- Sodium: 0 mg

Number of Servings: 4

Cooking Time: 30 minutes (plus chilling and freezing time)

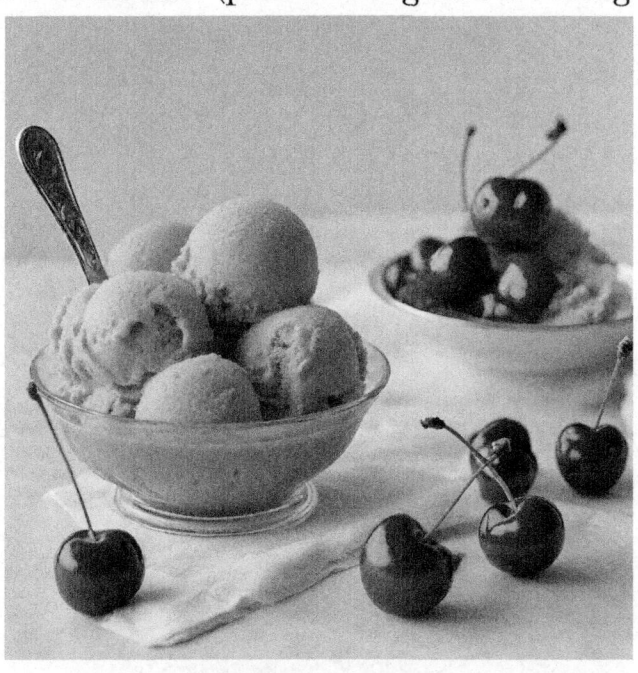

7. Pineapple Upside Down Cake

Ingredients:
- 1/4 cup butter
- 2/3 cup brown sugar
- 1 can (20 oz) pineapple slices, juice reserved
- 10 maraschino cherries
- 1 1/3 cups all-purpose flour
- 2/3 cup granulated sugar
- 2 teaspoons baking powder
- 1/4 teaspoon salt
- 1/3 cup vegetable oil
- 1 egg
- 1 teaspoon vanilla extract

Instructions:
1. Preheat oven to 350°F (175°C). Place butter in a 9-inch round cake pan and melt in the oven.
2. Sprinkle brown sugar evenly over melted butter. Arrange pineapple slices and cherries on the sugar.
3. In a bowl, mix flour, granulated sugar, baking powder, and salt. Add oil, egg, vanilla, and reserved pineapple juice. Beat until smooth.
4. Pour batter over pineapple and cherries in the pan.
5. Bake for 35-40 minutes, until a toothpick inserted into the center comes out clean.
6. Cool in the pan for 10 minutes, then invert onto a serving plate. Serve warm or at room temperature.

Nutritional Information (per serving):
- Calories: 330
- Protein: 3 g
- Carbohydrates: 50 g
- Fat: 14 g
- Fiber: 1 g
- Sodium: 220 mg

Number of Servings: 8
Cooking Time: 1 hour

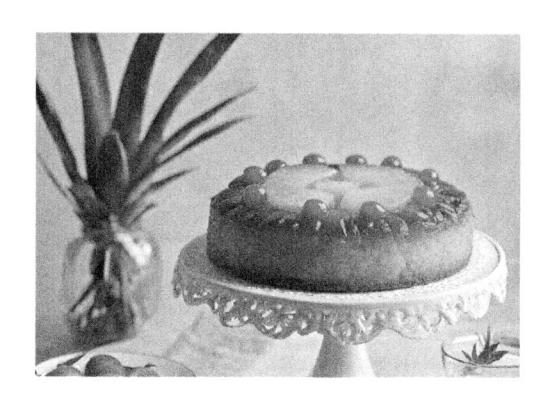

8. Coconut Macaroons

Ingredients:
- 3 cups shredded coconut
- 4 large egg whites
- 1/2 cup sugar
- 1 teaspoon vanilla extract
- 1/4 teaspoon salt

Instructions:
1. Preheat oven to 325°F (165°C). Line a baking sheet with parchment paper.
2. In a large bowl, whisk together egg whites, sugar, vanilla extract, and salt until the sugar is mostly dissolved.
3. Stir in the shredded coconut until well combined.
4. Drop tablespoonfuls of the mixture onto the prepared baking sheet, forming small mounds.
5. Bake for 20-25 minutes, or until the macaroons are golden brown.
6. Allow to cool on the baking sheet for 10 minutes before transferring to a wire rack to cool completely.

Nutritional Information (per serving):
- Calories: 130
- Protein: 2 g
- Carbohydrates: 15 g
- Fat: 7 g
- Fiber: 2 g
- Sodium: 75 mg

Number of Servings: 18
Cooking Time: 45 minutes

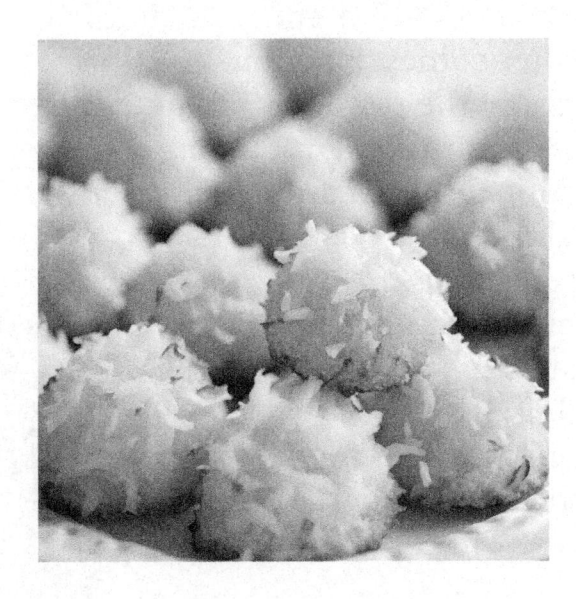

9. Orange Flavored Ricotta Cheesecake

Ingredients:
- 2 cups ricotta cheese
- 1/2 cup sugar
- Zest of 1 orange
- 2 eggs
- 1/2 teaspoon vanilla extract
- 1/4 cup all-purpose flour

Instructions:
1. Preheat oven to 350°F (175°C). Grease a 9-inch springform pan.
2. In a blender, combine ricotta cheese, sugar, orange zest, eggs, and vanilla extract until smooth.
3. Add flour and blend until just combined.
4. Pour the mixture into the prepared pan and smooth the top with a spatula.
5. Bake for 45-50 minutes, or until the center is set and the edges are lightly golden.
6. Let cool in the pan, then refrigerate for at least 4 hours before serving.

Nutritional Information (per serving):
- Calories: 160
- Protein: 7 g
- Carbohydrates: 15 g
- Fat: 8 g
- Fiber: 0 g
- Sodium: 60 mg

Number of Servings: 8

Cooking Time: 1 hour 10 minutes

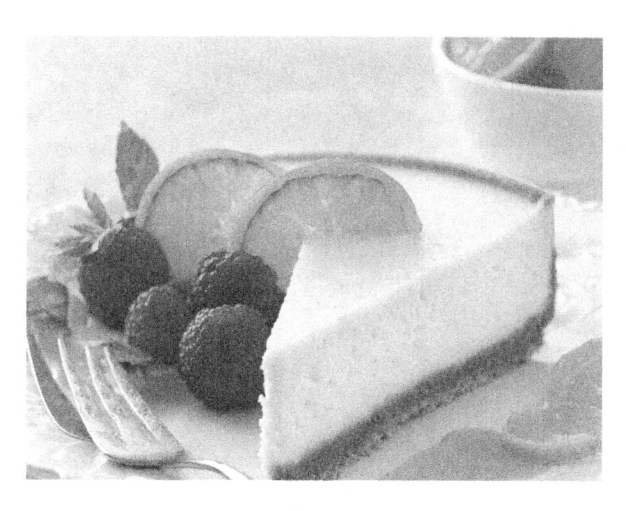

10. Fig and Honey Yogurt

Ingredients:
- 2 cups Greek yogurt
- 1/2 cup dried figs, chopped
- 2 tablespoons honey
- 1/2 teaspoon cinnamon

Instructions:
1. In a bowl, combine Greek yogurt, chopped figs, honey, and cinnamon.
2. Mix thoroughly until all ingredients are well combined.
3. Serve immediately or refrigerate for later.

Nutritional Information (per serving):
- Calories: 200
- Protein: 12 g
- Carbohydrates: 30 g
- Fat: 4 g
- Fiber: 2 g
- Sodium: 45 mg

Number of Servings: 4
Cooking Time: 10 minutes

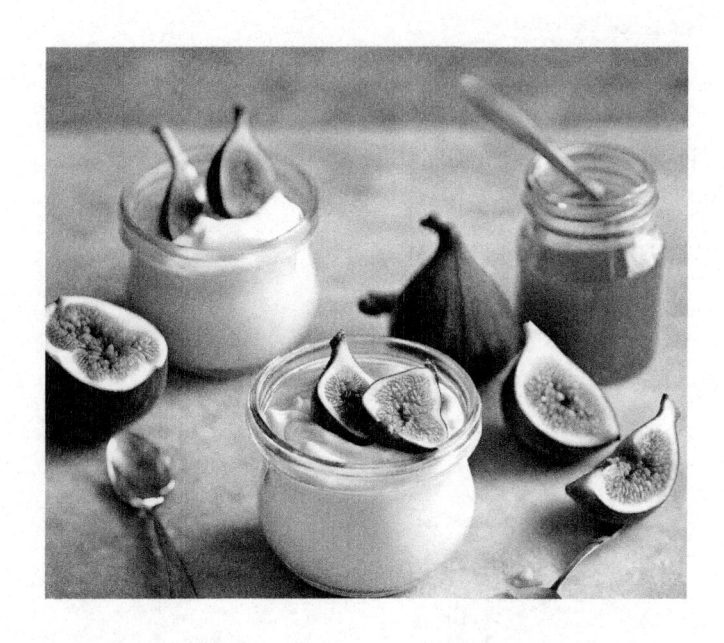

11. Raspberry Almond Bars

Ingredients:
- 1 cup all-purpose flour
- 1/4 cup sugar
- 1/2 cup butter, cold
- 1 cup raspberry jam
- 1/2 cup sliced almonds

Instructions:
1. Preheat oven to 350°F (175°C). Grease a 9x9 inch baking pan.
2. In a bowl, mix flour and sugar. Cut in butter until mixture resembles coarse crumbs.
3. Press two-thirds of the crumb mixture into the bottom of the prepared pan.
4. Spread the raspberry jam over the crust, then sprinkle with the remaining crumb mixture and sliced almonds.
5. Bake for 35-40 minutes, or until lightly golden.
6. Cool completely before cutting into bars.

Nutritional Information (per serving):
- Calories: 270
- Protein: 3 g
- Carbohydrates: 40 g
- Fat: 12 g
- Fiber: 2 g
- Sodium: 85 mg

Number of Servings: 12
Cooking Time: 55 minutes

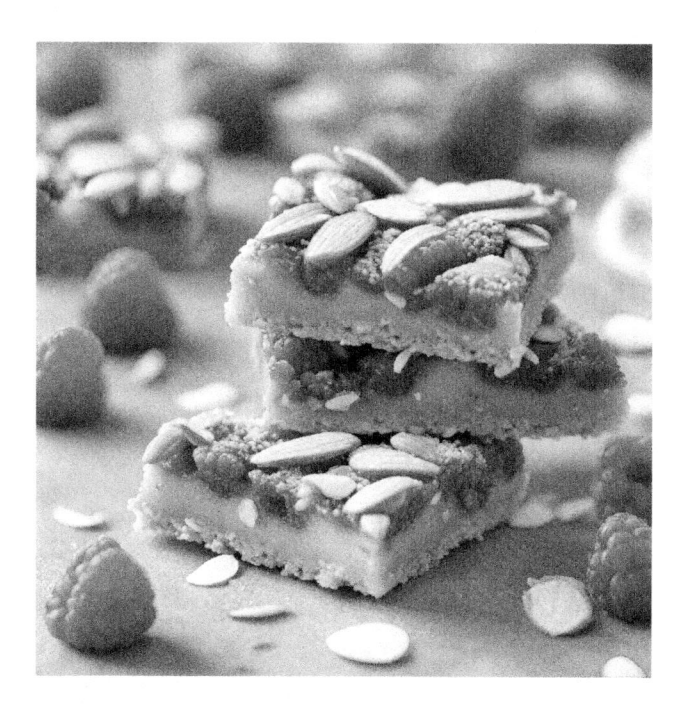

12. Strawberry Kiwi Fruit Tart

Ingredients:
- 1 pre-baked 9-inch tart shell
- 1 cup Greek yogurt
- 2 tablespoons honey
- 1 teaspoon vanilla extract
- 3 kiwis, peeled and sliced
- 1 cup strawberries, sliced
- 1/4 cup apricot jelly (optional, for glaze)

Instructions:
1. In a bowl, mix Greek yogurt, honey, and vanilla extract until smooth.
2. Spread the yogurt mixture into the pre-baked tart shell.
3. Arrange kiwi and strawberry slices on top of the yogurt in a decorative pattern.
4. If using, warm the apricot jelly until liquefied and brush over the fruit for a glossy finish.
5. Refrigerate for at least 1 hour before serving to set the yogurt filling.

Nutritional Information (per serving):
- Calories: 190
- Protein: 5 g
- Carbohydrates: 28 g
- Fat: 7 g
- Fiber: 2 g
- Sodium: 45 mg

Number of Servings: 8
Cooking Time: 1 hour 15 minutes (including refrigeration)

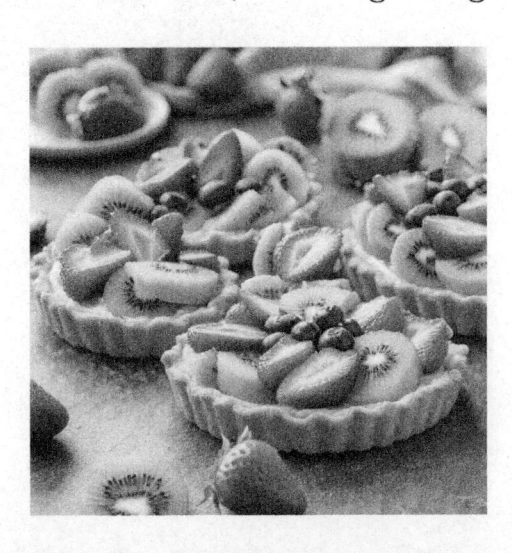

13. Berry Crisp with Oat Topping

Ingredients:
- 4 cups mixed berries (such as raspberries, blueberries, and blackberries)
- 1/4 cup sugar
- 1 tablespoon cornstarch
- **For the topping:**
  - 1/2 cup rolled oats
  - 1/4 cup flour
  - 1/4 cup brown sugar
  - 1/4 teaspoon cinnamon
  - 1/4 cup cold butter, cubed

Instructions:
1. Preheat oven to 375°F (190°C).
2. In a bowl, toss the berries with sugar and cornstarch, then pour into a greased 9-inch pie dish.
3. For the topping, in another bowl, mix oats, flour, brown sugar, and cinnamon. Rub in butter until the mixture is crumbly.
4. Sprinkle the oat topping over the berry mixture.
5. Bake for 35-40 minutes, until the topping is golden and the berries are bubbly.
6. Serve warm, ideally with a scoop of vanilla ice cream.

Nutritional Information (per serving):
- Calories: 250
- Protein: 2 g
- Carbohydrates: 38 g
- Fat: 10 g
- Fiber: 4 g
- Sodium: 60 mg

Number of Servings: 8
Cooking Time: 55 minutes

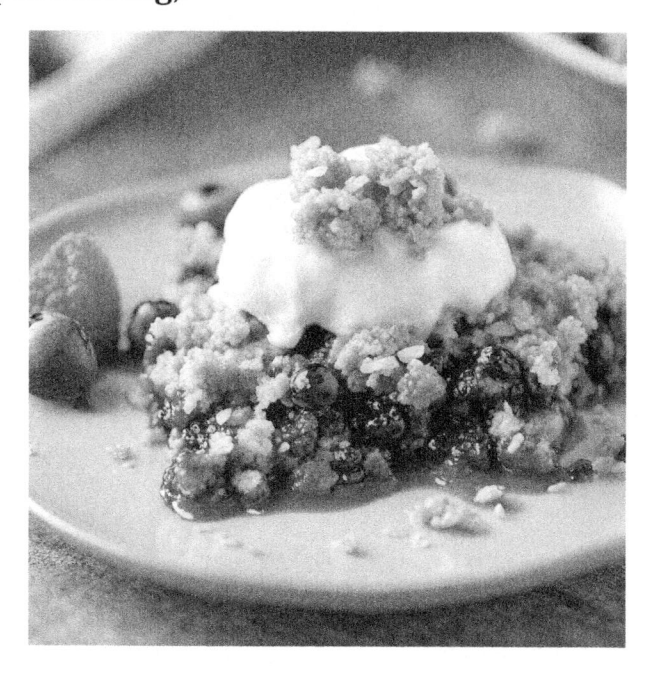

14. Carrot and Pineapple Cake

Ingredients:
- 2 cups all-purpose flour
- 2 teaspoons baking soda
- 1 teaspoon salt
- 2 teaspoons ground cinnamon
- 1 cup granulated sugar
- 1 cup vegetable oil
- 3 eggs
- 2 cups grated carrots
- 1 cup crushed pineapple, drained
- 1/2 cup chopped walnuts

Instructions:
1. Preheat oven to 350°F (175°C). Grease and flour a 9x13 inch baking pan.
2. In a bowl, mix flour, baking soda, salt, and cinnamon.
3. In another bowl, beat together sugar, oil, and eggs until smooth.
4. Stir in flour mixture until blended. Fold in carrots, pineapple, and walnuts.
5. Pour batter into the prepared pan.
6. Bake for 45 minutes, or until a toothpick inserted into the center comes out clean.
7. Cool in the pan for 10 minutes, then turn out onto a wire rack to cool completely.

Nutritional Information (per serving):
- Calories: 340
- Protein: 4 g
- Carbohydrates: 40 g
- Fat: 19 g
- Fiber: 2 g
- Sodium: 430 mg

Number of Servings: 12
Cooking Time: 55 minutes

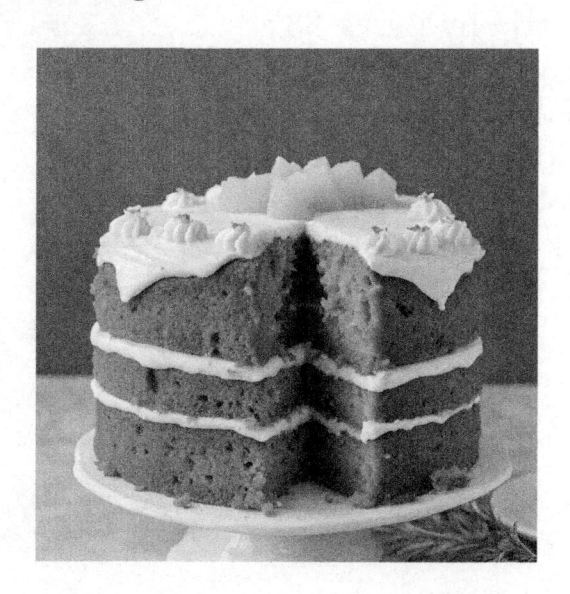

15. Blueberry Vanilla Yogurt Popsicles

Ingredients:
- 2 cups fresh blueberries
- 2 cups Greek yogurt
- 1/4 cup honey
- 1 teaspoon vanilla extract

Instructions:
1. In a blender, puree blueberries, yogurt, honey, and vanilla extract until smooth.
2. Pour the mixture into popsicle molds.
3. Freeze for at least 4 hours, or until firm.
4. Run warm water over the molds to release the popsicles before serving.

Nutritional Information (per serving):
- Calories: 150
- Protein: 5 g
- Carbohydrates: 25 g
- Fat: 2 g
- Fiber: 2 g
- Sodium: 35 mg

Number of Servings: 8
Cooking Time: 4 hours (freezing time)

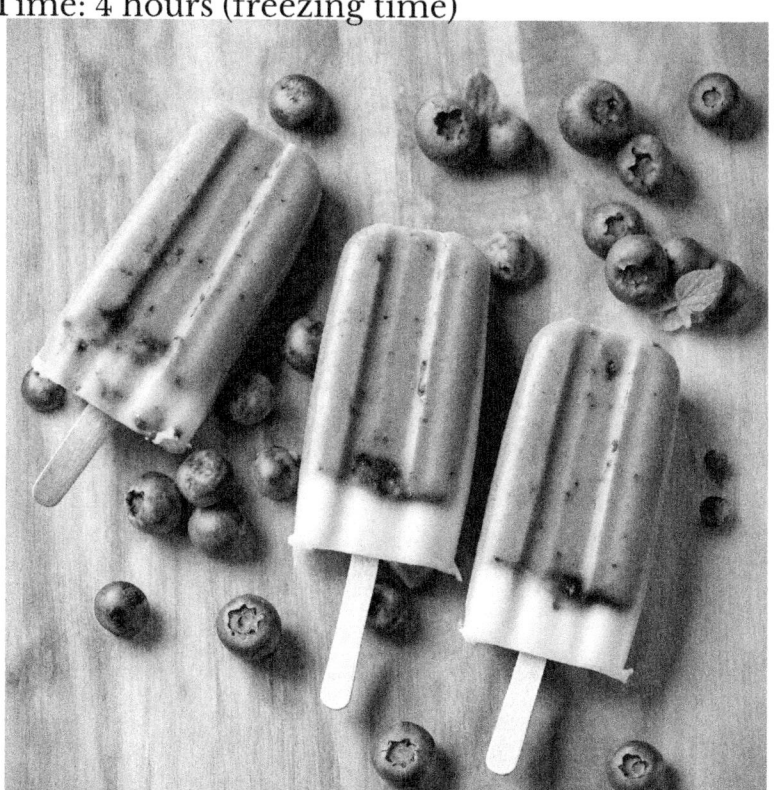

8-WEEK MEAL PLAN

Week 1
Day 1:
- **Breakfast**: Low-Oxalate Berry Smoothie
- **Lunch**: Chicken Caesar Salad
- **Dinner**: Grilled Halibut with Lemon Herb Sauce
- **Snack**: Greek Yogurt with Honey

Day 2:
- **Breakfast**: Banana Nut Muffins
- **Lunch**: Quinoa Tabbouleh
- **Dinner**: Baked Trout with Fennel and Citrus Salad
- **Snack**: Apple Slices with Almond Butter

Day 3:
- **Breakfast**: Cauliflower Hash Browns
- **Lunch**: Turkey and Avocado Wrap
- **Dinner**: Roasted Chicken with Root Vegetables
- **Snack**: Carrot Sticks with Hummus

Day 4:
- **Breakfast**: Oatmeal with Fresh Berries
- **Lunch**: Vegetable Stir-Fry with Tofu
- **Dinner**: Pasta Primavera with Whole Wheat Spaghetti
- **Snack**: Pear Slices

Day 5:
- **Breakfast**: Greek Yogurt Parfait
- **Lunch**: Beetroot and Goat Cheese Salad
- **Dinner**: Baked Tilapia with Lemon Parsley Quinoa
- **Snack**: Cucumber Slices with Low-fat Dip

Day 6:
- **Breakfast**: Scrambled Eggs with Spinach and Mushrooms
- **Lunch**: Lentil Soup
- **Dinner**: Grilled Salmon with Asparagus
- **Snack**: Fresh Pineapple Chunks

Day 7:
- **Breakfast**: Avocado Toast with Radish
- **Lunch**: Caprese Sandwich
- **Dinner**: Vegetarian Chili
- **Snack**: Blueberries and a Handful of Walnuts

Week 2

Day 8:
- **Breakfast**: Apple Cinnamon Oatmeal
- **Lunch**: Greek Yogurt Chicken Salad
- **Dinner**: Stir-Fried Beef and Broccoli
- **Snack**: Peach Slices

Day 9:
- **Breakfast**: Smoothie with Spinach, Kiwi, and Protein Powder
- **Lunch**: Balsamic Glazed Salmon
- **Dinner**: Turkey Meatloaf
- **Snack**: Low-Oxalate Nuts

Day 10:
- **Breakfast**: Cottage Cheese with Pineapple
- **Lunch**: Rice Noodle Salad with Peanut Dressing
- **Dinner**: Ratatouille
- **Snack**: Cherry Tomatoes

Day 11:
- **Breakfast**: Poached Eggs on Whole-Grain Toast
- **Lunch**: Roasted Turkey Breast Sandwich
- **Dinner**: Lemon Garlic Shrimp with Asparagus
- **Snack**: Mixed Berry Cup

Day 12:
- **Breakfast**: Banana Pancakes with Maple Syrup
- **Lunch**: Couscous with Roasted Vegetables
- **Dinner**: Cauliflower Steak with Tahini Sauce
- **Snack**: Apple and Walnut Salad

Day 13:
- **Breakfast**: Chia Seed Pudding
- **Lunch**: Vegetable Paella
- **Dinner**: Herbed Lamb Chops with Spinach Salad
- **Snack**: Mango Cubes

Day 14:
- **Breakfast**: Ricotta Pancakes
- **Lunch**: Moroccan Spiced Carrot Soup
- **Dinner**: Cod with Parsley Pesto and Steamed Vegetables
- **Snack**: Orange Segments

Week 3

Day 15:
- **Breakfast**: French Toast with Strawberries
- **Lunch**: Tofu and Vegetable Curry
- **Dinner**: Basil Pesto Pasta with Chicken
- **Snack**: Greek Yogurt with Mixed Nuts

Day 16:
- **Breakfast**: Vegetable Frittata
- **Lunch**: Stuffed Bell Peppers
- **Dinner**: Roasted Duck with Orange Sauce
- **Snack**: Kiwi Fruit

Day 17:
- **Breakfast**: Muesli with Skim Milk
- **Lunch**: Asian Cabbage Salad
- **Dinner**: Spaghetti Squash with Tomato Basil Sauce
- **Snack**: Pear and Cheese Plate

Day 18:
- **Breakfast**: Pumpkin Spice Smoothie
- **Lunch**: Tomato Basil Soup
- **Dinner**: Minted Pea and Barley Risotto
- **Snack**: Pomegranate Seeds

Day 19:
- **Breakfast**: Almond Butter and Banana Smoothie
- **Lunch**: Asian Glazed Salmon
- **Dinner**: Chickpea and Spinach Stew
- **Snack**: Cottage Cheese with Sliced Peaches

Day 20:
- **Breakfast**: Buckwheat Pancakes with Blueberries
- **Lunch**: Grilled Shrimp and Polenta
- **Dinner**: Cauliflower and Turmeric Soup
- **Snack**: Sliced Apples with Peanut Butter

Day 21:
- **Breakfast**: Cornflakes with Milk
- **Lunch**: Lemon Rosemary Grilled Swordfish
- **Dinner**: Zucchini Lasagna
- **Snack**: Frozen Grapes

Week 4

Day 22:
- **Breakfast**: Pear and Ricotta Cheese Toast
- **Lunch**: Smoked Salmon Salad with Cucumber and Dill
- **Dinner**: Garlic Herb Roasted Turkey
- **Snack**: Vanilla Greek Yogurt

Day 23:
- **Breakfast**: Smoothie with Papaya, Pineapple, and Protein Powder
- **Lunch**: Cold Noodle Salad with Sesame Dressing
- **Dinner**: Beef Stir-fry with Snap Peas and Mushrooms
- **Snack**: Carrot and Celery Sticks with Dip

Day 24:
- **Breakfast**: Omelette with Asparagus and Feta Cheese
- **Lunch**: Shrimp and Avocado Salad
- **Dinner**: Baked Lemon Pepper Cod
- **Snack**: Fresh Orange Slices

Day 25:
- **Breakfast**: Blueberry Almond Oatmeal
- **Lunch**: Tuna Salad Stuffed Avocado
- **Dinner**: Vegetarian Tacos with Cauliflower and Black Beans
- **Snack**: Sliced Bell Peppers with Hummus

Day 26:
- **Breakfast**: Coconut Yogurt with Kiwi and Pine Nuts
- **Lunch**: Barley and Roasted Vegetable Salad
- **Dinner**: Grilled Lamb with Mint Yogurt
- **Snack**: Apple with Almond Butter

Day 27:
- **Breakfast**: Quinoa Breakfast Bowl with Cherries and Pecans
- **Lunch**: Falafel Salad with Tahini Dressing
- **Dinner**: Chicken Tikka Masala with Basmati Rice
- **Snack**: Peach Slices

Day 28:
- **Breakfast**: Toasted English Muffin with Honey and Banana
- **Lunch**: Grilled Portobello Mushrooms with Arugula Salad
- **Dinner**: Pork Tenderloin with Apples and Onions
- **Snack**: Cottage Cheese with Raspberry Compote

Week 5

Day 29:
- **Breakfast**: Spinach and Mushroom Crepes
- **Lunch**: Chicken Waldorf Salad
- **Dinner**: Tilapia en Papillote with Zucchini and Bell Pepper
- **Snack**: Pineapple Chunks

Day 30:
- **Breakfast**: Avocado and Egg Breakfast Pizza
- **Lunch**: Cold Beet and Orange Salad
- **Dinner**: Moroccan Lamb Stew
- **Snack**: Greek Yogurt with Sliced Almonds

Day 31:
- **Breakfast**: Sweet Potato Pancakes
- **Lunch**: Soba Noodle Bowl with Edamame and Cucumber
- **Dinner**: Roasted Duck Breasts with Cherry Sauce
- **Snack**: Watermelon Salad with Mint

Day 32:
- **Breakfast**: Multigrain Porridge with Dried Apricots and Sunflower Seeds
- **Lunch**: Seared Scallops over Microgreens
- **Dinner**: Pork Chops with Sauteed Apples and Brussels Sprouts
- **Snack**: Orange and Kiwi Fruit Salad

Day 33:
- **Breakfast**: Protein-Packed Smoothie Bowl
- **Lunch**: Quiche with Tomato and Spinach
- **Dinner**: Spiced Chicken with Couscous
- **Snack**: Banana and Cottage Cheese

Day 34:
- **Breakfast**: Muesli with Skim Milk and Dried Cranberries
- **Lunch**: Spicy Tofu Lettuce Wraps
- **Dinner**: Italian Baked Fish with Olives and Capers
- **Snack**: Pear and Cottage Cheese

Day 35:
- **Breakfast**: Cheddar and Broccoli Frittata
- **Lunch**: Asian Chicken Salad with Mandarin Oranges
- **Dinner**: Vegetable Lasagna with Spinach and Ricotta
- **Snack**: Mixed Nuts

Week 6

Day 36:
- **Breakfast**: Poached Eggs with Avocado and Whole-Grain Toast
- **Lunch**: Nicoise Salad with Tuna
- **Dinner**: Grilled Swordfish with Mango Salsa
- **Snack**: Baked Apple with Cinnamon

Day 37:
- **Breakfast**: Cottage Cheese Pancakes with Blueberry Compote
- **Lunch**: Mediterranean Chickpea Wrap
- **Dinner**: Thai Basil Chicken
- **Snack**: Fresh Figs with Honey

Day 38:
- **Breakfast**: French Toast with Prunes and Maple Syrup
- **Lunch**: Salmon Nicoise Platter
- **Dinner**: Italian Stuffed Bell Peppers
- **Snack**: Kiwi and Strawberry Salad

Day 39:
- **Breakfast**: Almond and Banana Smoothie
- **Lunch**: Vegetable and Bean Burrito
- **Dinner**: Garlic Butter Shrimp with Asparagus
- **Snack**: Pomegranate Seeds

Day 40:
- **Breakfast**: Oat Bran Muffins with Apple Sauce
- **Lunch**: Turkey and Swiss Cheese Roll-Ups
- **Dinner**: Vegan Mushroom Stroganoff
- **Snack**: Melon Balls

Day 41:
- **Breakfast**: Pineapple and Coconut Oatmeal
- **Lunch**: Greek Salad with Chicken
- **Dinner**: Seared Tuna Steak with Olive Tapenade
- **Snack**: Fresh Pear Slices

Day 42:
- **Breakfast**: Egg White Scramble with Fresh Herbs
- **Lunch**: Roast Beef and Arugula Sandwich
- **Dinner**: Veggie Stir-Fry with Tofu
- **Snack**: Yogurt with Pumpkin Seeds

Week 7

Day 43:
- **Breakfast**: Cinnamon Pear Oatmeal
- **Lunch**: Crab Salad with Mixed Greens
- **Dinner**: Lemon and Herb Baked Snapper
- **Snack**: Non-fat Plain Yogurt with a drizzle of Honey

Day 44:
- **Breakfast**: Egg Muffins with Kale and Red Peppers
- **Lunch**: Spicy Grilled Shrimp Tacos
- **Dinner**: Moroccan Vegetable Tagine
- **Snack**: Sliced Cucumbers with Low-Fat Ranch Dressing

Day 45:
- **Breakfast**: Butternut Squash and Apple Hash
- **Lunch**: Quinoa Salad with Lemon and Herbs
- **Dinner**: Roasted Chicken with Thyme and Onions
- **Snack**: Fresh Mango Slices

Day 46:
- **Breakfast**: Greek Yogurt with Peach Compote
- **Lunch**: Tuna Niçoise Salad
- **Dinner**: Beef Stroganoff with Mushrooms
- **Snack**: A handful of Mixed Berries

Day 47:
- **Breakfast**: Toasted Bagel with Avocado Spread
- **Lunch**: Lentil and Vegetable Stew
- **Dinner**: Pork Loin with Roasted Apples and Parsnips
- **Snack**: A small bowl of Cherries

Day 48:
- **Breakfast**: Berry and Flaxseed Smoothie
- **Lunch**: Chicken and Avocado Wrap
- **Dinner**: Cod with Tomato and Olive Tapenade
- **Snack**: Air-popped Popcorn

Day 49:
- **Breakfast**: Omelette with Asparagus and Goat Cheese
- **Lunch**: Beet and Citrus Salad
- **Dinner**: Vegetarian Paella
- **Snack**: A bowl of Pineapple and Kiwi

Week 8

Day 50:
- **Breakfast**: Carrot and Ginger Juice, Whole Wheat Toast
- **Lunch**: Smoked Salmon and Cream Cheese Bagel
- **Dinner**: Thai Green Curry with Tofu
- **Snack**: Fresh Apple Slices with Peanut Butter

Day 51:
- **Breakfast**: Coconut Milk Porridge with Banana
- **Lunch**: Greek Orzo Salad
- **Dinner**: Baked Haddock with Sweet Potato Wedges
- **Snack**: A handful of Almonds

Day 52:
- **Breakfast**: Mixed Berry Parfait with Granola
- **Lunch**: Spinach and Feta Stuffed Chicken Breast
- **Dinner**: Vegan Chili
- **Snack**: Celery Sticks with Almond Butter

Day 53:
- **Breakfast**: Sweet Corn and Zucchini Fritters
- **Lunch**: Shrimp and Pineapple Salad
- **Dinner**: Lamb Kebabs with Mint Yogurt Sauce
- **Snack**: A small bowl of Watermelon

Day 54:
- **Breakfast**: Banana and Walnut Bread
- **Lunch**: Caprese Salad with Balsamic Glaze
- **Dinner**: Chicken Marsala
- **Snack**: Sliced Peaches

Day 55:
- **Breakfast**: Almond Butter and Banana Smoothie
- **Lunch**: Kale and Quinoa Salad with Lemon Vinaigrette
- **Dinner**: Grilled Swordfish with Lemon and Dill
- **Snack**: Greek Yogurt with a sprinkle of Cinnamon

Day 56:
- **Breakfast**: Scrambled Eggs with Tomato and Chives
- **Lunch**: Roasted Eggplant Sandwich
- **Dinner**: Turkey Burgers with Sweet Potato Fries
- **Snack**: Mixed Nuts

FOOD TRACKER JOURNAL

Write down everything you ate and drank yesterday. Highlight any items you know are high in sodium, oxalates, or protein.

FLUID INTAKE

FOODS TO AVOID

DAYS	BREAKFAST	LUNCH	DINNER
MON			
TUE			
WED			
THU			
FRI			
SAT			
SUN			

FOOD TRACKER JOURNAL

What are your go-to snacks and meals on a typical day? Identify which of these might be high in oxalates or sodium.

FLUID INTAKE

◊ ◊ ◊ ◊ ◊ ◊ ◊
◊ ◊ ◊ ◊ ◊ ◊ ◊
◊ ◊ ◊ ◊ ◊ ◊ ◊

FOODS TO AVOID

DAYS	BREAKFAST	LUNCH	DINNER
MON			
TUE			
WED			
THU			
FRI			
SAT			
SUN			

FOOD TRACKER JOURNAL

How much water do you typically drink in a day? Set a goal for increasing your water intake to help prevent future kidney stones.

WATER INTAKE

FOODS TO AVOID

DAYS	BREAKFAST	LUNCH	DINNER
MON			
TUE			
WED			
THU			
FRI			
SAT			
SUN			

FOOD TRACKER JOURNAL

List all sources of calcium in your diet. How can you balance your calcium intake with oxalate-rich foods to reduce stone risk?

_____
_____
_____
_____
_____
_____
_____
_____

WATER INTAKE

◊ ◊ ◊ ◊ ◊ ◊ ◊
◊ ◊ ◊ ◊ ◊ ◊ ◊
◊ ◊ ◊ ◊ ◊ ◊ ◊

FOODS TO AVOID

_____
_____
_____
_____
_____
_____
_____

DAYS	BREAKFAST	LUNCH	DINNER
MON			
TUE			
WED			
THU			
FRI			
SAT			
SUN			

FOOD TRACKER JOURNAL

Find three packaged foods in your home and write down their sodium content. How could you find lower-sodium alternatives?

WATER INTAKE

FOODS TO AVOID

DAYS	BREAKFAST	LUNCH	DINNER
MON			
TUE			
WED			
THU			
FRI			
SAT			
SUN			

FOOD TRACKER JOURNAL

Think about the last time you ate out. What could you have chosen differently to adhere to a kidney stone diet?

WATER INTAKE

○ ○ ○ ○ ○ ○ ○
○ ○ ○ ○ ○ ○ ○
○ ○ ○ ○ ○ ○ ○

FOODS TO AVOID

DAYS	BREAKFAST	LUNCH	DINNER
MON			
TUE			
WED			
THU			
FRI			
SAT			
SUN			

FOOD TRACKER JOURNAL

Note any symptoms or discomfort you experience daily. Can you identify any links between your symptoms and your eating habits?

WATER INTAKE

◊ ◊ ◊ ◊ ◊ ◊ ◊
◊ ◊ ◊ ◊ ◊ ◊ ◊
◊ ◊ ◊ ◊ ◊ ◊ ◊

FOODS TO AVOID

DAYS	BREAKFAST	LUNCH	DINNER
MON			
TUE			
WED			
THU			
FRI			
SAT			
SUN			

FOOD TRACKER JOURNAL

Who in your life can help you stay committed to your new diet? How will you engage them in your process?

WATER INTAKE

FOODS TO AVOID

DAYS	BREAKFAST	LUNCH	DINNER
MON			
TUE			
WED			
THU			
FRI			
SAT			
SUN			

FOOD TRACKER JOURNAL

At the end of each week, reflect on your dietary adherence. What were your successes and challenges? How can you improve next week?

....
....
....
....
....
....
....

WATER INTAKE

○ ○ ○ ○ ○ ○ ○
○ ○ ○ ○ ○ ○ ○
○ ○ ○ ○ ○ ○ ○

FOODS TO AVOID

_____
_____
_____
_____
_____
_____
_____

DAYS	BREAKFAST	LUNCH	DINNER
MON			
TUE			
WED			
THU			
FRI			
SAT			
SUN			

Scan the QR code below to get a surprise bonus!